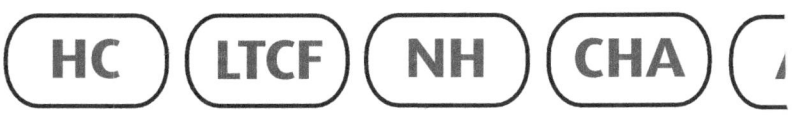

interRAI Clinical Assessment Protocols (CAPs)

For Use with Community and Long-Term Care Assessment Instruments*

Version 9.1

interRAI Instrument and Systems Development Committee

John N. Morris, PhD, MSW [Chair]
Katherine Berg, PhD, PT
Magnus Björkgren, PhD
Harriet Finne-Soveri, MD, PhD
Brant E. Fries, PhD
Dinnus Frijters, PhD
Ruedi Gilgen, MD
Len Gray, MD, PhD

Catherine Hawes, PhD
Jean-Claude Henrard, MD
John P. Hirdes, PhD
Gunnar Ljunggren, MD, PhD
Sue Nonemaker, RN, MS
Knight Steel, MD
Katarzyna Szczerbińska, MD, PhD

Additional authors and members of a special interRAI CAP development support committee

Pauline Belleville-Taylor, RN, MS, CS
Terry Rabinowitz, MD
Trevor Frise Smith, PhD

John N. Morris, PhD, MSW
Brant E. Fries, PhD
John P. Hirdes, PhD

*Applicable assessment instruments include the Resident Assessment Instrument (RAI) MDS 2.0 for nursing homes, RAI-Home Care (RAI-HC), interRAI Long-Term Care Facilities (LTCF), interRAI Home Care (HC), interRAI Community Health Assessment (CHA), and interRAI Assisted Living (AL)

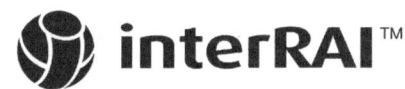

www.interRAI.org

Version 9.1.2 interRAI Standard Edition

Library of Congress Cataloging-in-Publication Data
InterRAI clinical assessment protocols (CAPs) for use with community and long-term care assessment instruments / interRAI Instrument and Systems Development Committee ; John N. Morris . . . [et al.].—Version 9.1.
    p. ; cm.
    Other title: Clinical assessment protocols (CAPs) for use with community and long-term care assessment instruments
    Includes bibliographical references.
    Summary: "interRAI Clinical Assessment Protocols are designed to assist the assessor to interpret systematically all the information recorded on its assessment instruments for home care, community health, long-term care facilities, and assisted living"—Provided by publisher.
    ISBN 978-1-936065-15-8
    1. Medical care—Evaluation. 2. Medical protocols. 3. Long-term care facilities. 4. Community health services. 5. Nursing assessment. I. Morris, John N. (John Norman), 1941– II. interRAI (Organization). Instrument and Systems Development Committee. III. Title: Clinical assessment protocols (CAPs) for use with community and long-term care assessment instruments.
    [DNLM: 1. Home Care Services—organization & administration. 2. Health Services for the Aged—organization & administration. 3. Long-Term Care—organization & administration. 4. Needs Assessment. WY 115 I615 2010]

    RA399.A3I58 2010
    362.1068--dc22

                          2010023168

interRAI publications packaged by Open Book Systems (OBS), Inc.
Rockport, Massachusetts, USA
www.obs.com

Suggested Citation
Morris JN, Berg K, Björkgren M, Finne-Soveri H, Fries BE, Frijters D, Gilgen R, Gray L, Hawes C, Henrard JC, Hirdes JP, Ljunggren G, Nonemaker S, Steel K, Szczerbińska K, Belleville-Taylor P, Rabinowitz T, Smith TF. interRAI Clinical Assessment Protocols (CAPs) for Use with Community and Long-Term Care Assessment Instruments. Version 9.1. Washington, DC: interRAI, 2010.

Acknowledgments

interRAI acknowledges the important contribution and support of Hebrew SeniorLife in Boston, and most especially the contribution of the support staff at the Institute for Aging Research.

For information or comments on interRAI and its assessment instruments, visit www.interRAI.org

Disclaimer

Licensing interRAI Assessment Systems

Preface

The New Generation of interRAI Clinical Assessment Protocols

As part of a multiyear initiative to update its entire family of assessment instruments, interRAI is pleased to release new Clinical Assessment Protocols (CAPs) for use with its assessment instruments for home care, community health, long-term care facilities, and assisted living. The new CAPs can also be used with the prior generation of interRAI assessment instruments used in long-term care facilities [also referred to as nursing homes] (the MDS 2.0) and home care (the HC 2.0). As a result, we hope clinicians using either the prior instruments or the new suite of instruments will be able to benefit from this major research initiative.

This set of twenty-seven new CAPs was first released at the joint interRAI-Canadian Institute for Health Information conference held in Ottawa, Canada in May 2007. New CAPs for use with interRAI's inpatient psychiatry and community mental health instruments (interRAI Mental Health and interRAI Community Mental Health) will be released mid-late 2010. Three working groups are also in the process of developing the first generation of CAPs for the interRAI Acute Care (mid-late 2010 release), interRAI Palliative Care (mid-late 2010 release), and interRAI Intellectual Disability (2011 release) instruments.

The effort to develop the new CAPs was led by interRAI's Instrument and Systems Development (ISD) committee chaired by John Morris, PhD, MSW. The ISD and support subcommittee membership comprises a multidisciplinary team from nine countries, including

Australia	Len Gray, MD, PhD
Canada	Katherine Berg, PhD, PT; John P. Hirdes, PhD; Trevor Frise Smith, PhD
Finland	Magnus Björkgren, PhD; Harriet Finne-Soveri, MD, PhD
France	Jean-Claude Henrard, MD
Netherlands	Dinnus Frijters, PhD
Poland	Katarzyna Szczerbińska, MD, PhD
Sweden	Gunnar Ljunggren, MD, PhD
Switzerland	Ruedi Gilgen, MD
United States	Pauline Belleville Taylor, RN, MS, CS; Brant E. Fries, PhD; Catherine Hawes, PhD; John N. Morris, PhD, MSW; Knight Steel, MD; Sue Nonemaker, RN, MS; Terry Rabinowitz, MD

In addition, members of the ISD committee and its subcommittees have engaged in an extensive consultation effort to obtain feedback from stakeholders including frontline clinicians and researchers from around the globe. In the United States, clinicians from the Hebrew SeniorLife at Boston reviewed the draft CAPs. In Canada, the Canadian Institute for Health Information (CIHI), with coordination by Nancy Curtin-Telegdi, MA, Nancy White, MBA, and care professionals from across the country, provided substantial feedback on the draft CAPs.

Developing these new CAPs involved a comprehensive research effort that considered the most current evidence from the peer-reviewed literature, international best practice guidelines, and information provided by subject matter experts from around the globe. A particularly important feature of this work was the extensive use of interRAI's large data holdings from Canada, United States, eleven European countries, and Hong Kong to redefine the CAP triggers and to test the factors associated with differential outcomes of care. interRAI was also able to draw on several private research data files maintained by members from Canada and the United States. For example, Canadian and European data on over one-half million home care assessments were analyzed to evaluate home care outcomes. Similarly, over 300,000 Ontario complex continuing care (CCC) assessments and millions of assessments from U.S. nursing homes provided insights into the experience in long-term care facilities, skilled nursing facilities, and CCC hospitals/units. **The estimated percentage of persons given for each triggered CAP group is based on these data.**

The CAP redevelopment effort has been a massive international research undertaking that focused on improving the quality of care and quality of life of vulnerable populations. In combination with interRAI's release of a suite of twelve new versions of its assessment instruments, this work represents a major step forward in developing a truly integrated health information system.

Contents

Part IV   Clinical Issues CAPs   99

Appendices

Introduction: The interRAI CAPs

interRAI Assessment Instruments

The interRAI Clinical Assessment Protocols (CAPs) are designed to work with a variety of interRAI's community and long-term care assessment instruments. The released CAPs in this instructional manual support the following instruments:

- Nursing Home MDS (NH), Version 2.0 (MDS 2.0)

- RAI-Home Care (HC), Version 2.0 (HC 2.0)

- interRAI Long-Term Care Facilities (LTCF)

- interRAI Home Care (HC)

- interRAI Community Health Assessment (CHA)

- interRAI Assisted Living (AL)

In designing these instruments, interRAI strived to create user friendly, reliable, person-centered assessment systems that inform and guide comprehensive care and service planning in each of these settings and programs. The CAPs focus on a person's function and quality of life, assessing the person's needs, strengths, and preferences. They facilitate referrals when appropriate, and when used on multiple occasions, they provide the basis for an outcome-based assessment of the person's response to care or services.

interRAI CAPs Overview

interRAI's assessment instruments enable care providers to address key factors in the person's life, including aspects of function, health, social support, service use, and quality of life. Subsets of these items have been selected to identify persons who may benefit from care and support in each of the many problem areas referenced by the CAPs, with subsets of items forming CAP triggers. The CAP trigger items are thus referenced in the description of each CAP, and the Appendices reference how to secure the computer code used to formulate these CAP triggers. **As this manual addresses triggering for multiple instruments, an individual item referenced by a trigger may not appear in every instrument.**

The goals of care vary from one CAP to the next, but include the possibility of resolving the problem, reducing the risk of decline, or increasing the potential for improvement. These subsets of items, known as "CAP triggers," link the information gathered in the assessment to the basic problem referenced by the CAP. Compared to earlier versions of the CAP triggers, this triggering approach now seeks to identify two types of persons. First are those who have a higher than expected likelihood of declining — a very typical scenario, for example, for long-stay residents. Second are persons who have an increased likelihood of improving, including those declining due to a recent acute problem (for example, delirium, psychosis, falls, pneumonia) and whose symptoms will be alleviated when the problem is addressed. Using this approach, it was possible to cut the proportion of CAPs triggered for follow-up in all settings. For example, of the eighteen problem areas represented by the earlier MDS 2.0 versions of these CAPs, the trigger rate has dropped by one-half. Finally, interRAI is updating the approach to care instructions provided in each of these problem areas, focusing where possible on clinical issues and strategies that have been empirically demonstrated to lead to positive outcomes. We see this as a continuing effort to refine the guidelines as the quality of the data and knowledge — ours and others — improves. interRAI intends to continue to review these CAPs — both the text and the triggering logic — to update them to improve practice patterns.

For those triggered, each CAP contains care guidelines to help to think through the relevant underlying issues and move toward a plan of care. Clinical Assessment Protocols (CAPs) guide the plan of care to resolve problems, reduce the risk of decline, or increase the potential for improvement.

interRAI's CAPs cover problems in four broad areas:

- Functional performance

- Cognition and mental health

- Social life

- Clinical issues

Persons typically trigger on multiple CAPs, with the overall triggering rate determined by the vulnerability of the person and the setting in which he or she is seen.*

- Persons in North American nursing homes average 4 triggered CAPs (of 22 CAPs assessed).

- Persons screened for admission to North American nursing homes average 7 triggered CAPs (of 25 CAPs assessed using the interRAI Home Care form).

- Persons in home care programs that serve as an alternative to nursing home placement average 6.5 triggered CAPs (of the 25 assessed).

- Persons in a typical home care program in Canada, Europe, or Hong Kong average 5.5 triggered CAPs (of the 25 assessed).

- Even some independent older adults trigger on these CAPs, but the average is only about 2 CAPs per person, with over 75% of these persons having a problem on the Prevention CAP, and 15 to 20% having problems with social relationships, pain, falls, and mood.

The goal of the health care professional is to use the information provided in the CAP Guidelines to arrive at a plan of care, and where possible and required, provide the service or make an appropriate referral. At the same time, health care professionals may find themselves working within a context where reimbursement systems or eligibility requirements limit the care options. Thus, they may not be able to offer services to fully address the person's needs in all triggered problem areas at that point in time. Nevertheless, a comprehensive assessment that includes the strengths, preferences, and needs of the person can be useful to develop priorities, schedule services, make appropriate referrals, and assess program outcomes. The development of a care plan should be a collaborative effort between the health care team, the person, and his or her informal supporters. Whenever possible and appropriate, the preferences and priorities of the person should be the start-

*Throughout this manual the results of interRAI's analyses of data holdings from North America, Europe, and the Pacific Rim will be reported in relation to specific CAPs. The reported percentages arise from research undertaken specifically in support of the CAP redevelopment effort. A series of peer-reviewed publications that provide more detailed technical descriptions of this work is in preparation.

ing point for developing a care plan that builds on his or her strengths in order to address specific needs.

CAPs by setting: The following chart indicates where interRAI's CAPs are applied.

CAP	Home Care / Assisted Living	Community Health Assessment [note: all HC CAPs when functional supplement used]	Nursing Home / Long-Term Care Facility
FUNCTIONAL PERFORMANCE			
Physical Activities Promotion	X	X	X[a]
Instrumental Activities of Daily Living	X	X	
Activities of Daily Living	X	X	X
Home Environment Optimization	X[b]		
Institutional Risk	X		
Physical Restraints	X		X
COGNITION/ MENTAL HEALTH			
Cognitive Loss	X	X	X
Delirium	X		X
Communication	X	X	X
Mood	X	X	X
Behavior	X		X
Abusive Relationship	X	X	
SOCIAL LIFE			
Activities			X
Informal Support	X[b]	X	
Social Relationship	X	X	X
CLINICAL ISSUES[c]			
Falls	X	X	X
Pain	X	X	X
Pressure Ulcer	X		X
Cardiorespiratory Conditions	X	X	X
Undernutrition	X[d]		X
Dehydration	X[b]	X	X
Feeding Tube	X[b]		X
Prevention	X	X	X[e]
Appropriate Medications	X	X	X
Tobacco and Alcohol Use	X	X	X[f]
Urinary Incontinence	X	X	X
Bowel Conditions	X		X

[a] interRAI LTCF, not MDS 2.0.
[b] interRAI HC, not interRAI AL.
[c] The Cardiorespiratory and Appropriate Medications CAPs cannot be calculated for the abbreviated quarterly nursing home assessments.
[d] interRAI HC, not HC 2.0.
[e] Suite, not MDS 2.0.
[f] Suite, not MDS 2.0.

Part I

Functional Performance CAPs

1. Physical Activities Promotion CAP

2. Instrumental Activities of Daily Living CAP

3. Activities of Daily Living CAP

4. Home Environment Optimization CAP

5. Institutional Risk CAP

6. Physical Restraints CAP

Physical Activities Promotion CAP

Problem

The Physical Activities Promotion CAP identifies persons who engage in low levels of physical activity — that is, they engage in less than 2 hours of physical activity over a 3- day period (performing instrumental tasks around the home, walking, or carrying out a planned exercise program). At this level of engagement, most persons are at an elevated risk of having a number of health complications and physical decline.

The benefits of a more intensive schedule of physical activity include enhanced cardiovascular endurance, better mood, a lower risk of falling, a slowing of functional decline, and better control of weight. Persons who engage in higher levels of regular physical activity, such as walking, have been shown to have better balance, more mobility, and greater strength in their legs.

Frail persons residing in long-term care facilities may benefit as well from targeted exercise programs, with a resultant slowing in loss of abilities in everyday activities of daily life (for example, dressing and walking). Cognitively impaired persons may also benefit from increased physical activity and, as is true for everyone, they are more likely to participate in activities that they did before or that they currently enjoy. For example, persons who played golf may enjoy putting practice. Studies have shown benefits of walking programs in long-term care facilities, evening walking for wanderers, and multisensory exercise programs.

Achieving a consistent pattern of at least 1 hour of physical activity a day can be a challenge. Thus, for persons triggered by this CAP, one needs to follow a gradual four-step program: (1) educate the person about the benefits of higher levels of physical activity; (2) identify why the person has not been more active; (3) schedule a step-by-step program of physical activity acceptable to the person; and (4) encourage the person to gradually adopt and then continue with the physical activity program over an extended period of time.

Effective physical activity counseling programs assist the person in developing a concrete plan consistent with his or her goals, while providing acceptable strategies to overcome barriers. These barriers might include a lack of interest, the objection

Overall Goals of Care

- Increase hours of exercise and physical activity.

- Prevent loss of independent function in IADLs, ADLs, and mobility.

- Develop concrete goals and strategies to address potential barriers.

- Among the specific strategies to be considered, include the following: involvement in housework and shopping, mobility indoors and outdoors, increasing the distance walked (or wheeled), and increasing the speed of walking.

- For lower functioning persons, engage the family, staff, or caregivers in counseling activities and strategizing to overcome barriers.

of loved ones, an absence of time to engage in the activities, poor weather, fluctuating health status, unexpected health events that involve periods of bed rest or inactivity, or limitations due to a stroke or cognitive impairment that restricts either understanding or the ability to consistently follow through on the agreed plan. But regardless of the barriers, the goal of this CAP is to work with the person to find a suitable physical activity strategy that fits into his or her lifestyle.

Physical Activities Promotion CAP Trigger

The goal of this CAP is to increase physical activity levels of functionally capable sedentary adults. In order to be successful and appropriate, a plan to overcome medical barriers and conditions should be designed in collaboration with the person's physician.

TRIGGERED TO FACILITATE IMPROVEMENT

This subgroup is defined by two factors:

- First, the person is engaged in less than 2 hours of physical activity over the last 3 days.

- Second, the person has one or more of the following positive assets:

  - Moves in the residence without help or cueing

  - Goes up and down stairs without help

  - Believes he or she could be more independent

  - Caregiver believes the person could be more independent

  - The person has good prospects of recovery from current diseases or conditions

Given these functional reserves, persons in this subgroup are the most likely to be able to achieve increased hours of physical activity. Yet, only a small fraction of this population has been shown to improve (about 11%) over the following 90-day period, and the principal focus of care is to increase the likelihood of this happening. Note that this group includes about 30% of persons receiving home care, 25% of persons in long-term care facilities, and 15% of older adults living independently in the community.

NOT TRIGGERED   All other persons.

Physical Activities Promotion CAP Guidelines

Personal choice. To promote change in physical activity levels, it is essential to involve the person in choosing the goals and strategies to achieve the objectives. The aim of the professional working with the person is to

- Increase awareness of the health benefits of exercise.

- Help the person contemplate a future lifestyle in which exercise is a part of his or her weekly routine.

- Engage the person in a discussion of the types of exercise (such as activities around the house, walking, or dancing) that they had enjoyed previously or others they would like to try at this time.

- Discuss any barriers that might prevent the person from increasing his or her exercise levels or maintaining these levels. A low-key approach is most likely to be effective in increasing the person's (or family's) receptiveness and readiness to change.

Options for persons with high (good) functioning (both physical and cognitive). To determine the person's level of interest in exercise and physical activity, consider the following:

- Discuss the person's preferences for exercise such as dancing, walking as a part of daily life or as a planned activity (alone, with others, when doing certain activities, over a fixed course), bicycling, and exercise classes. Persons who previously enjoyed exercise are more likely to return to exercise.

- Discuss options to suit the person's interests and level of functioning.

- Identify the person's level of readiness for change.

  - The proposed activity should be realistic and accessible.

  - Selection of activities that are meaningful for the person are more likely to be followed.

  - A nonmotivated person may begin with small steps, for example, walking more frequently.

  - A sedentary person may benefit from a discussion of changes in his or her daily routines that promote lower levels of physical activity.

  - A person with little or no interest in exercise may be willing to discuss other goals and how exercise might assist in helping meet them.

  - For the motivated person, discuss how appropriate physical activities can become a part of the daily routine in addition to individually tailored training programs in the home or community.

- Some persons will need practical information on how to accomplish the goals given their current health status.

- When there is agreement on exercise goals, engage the person in a discussion of potential barriers that could interfere. For each barrier consider solutions.

- Provide as much information as possible about suitable and available programs.

  - For any age, exercise must be undertaken sensibly to avoid injury and complications. Therefore, it is necessary to consult and work collaboratively with the person's primary care physician and ensure that proper screening is performed before an exercise program begins.

  - Persons who are willing and able to attend community-based programs may be referred to them.

  - In some areas, programs are targeted to persons with specific chronic conditions, and some may offer special accommodations.

  - Family members or volunteers may be able to assist in outdoor activities if the person is not confident about walking outdoors.

  - Persons who do not wish to join exercise classes or group activities may use available home exercise videos.

- Develop a schedule of physical activity including

  - Aerobic activities, such as moderately intense walks for at least 30 minutes, 4 to 5 days a week.

  - Progressively more intense muscle strengthening exercises on at least 2 nonconsecutive days each week. Examples include progressive weight training and weight bearing calisthenics.

  - Flexibility training activities in conjunction with the muscle strengthening exercise routine.

  - Balance exercises several times a week.

Options for persons with IADL or ADL problems. If the person has triggered on either the IADL or ADL CAP, give precedence to those guidelines. Otherwise, consider the following:

- If the decline is recent, refer the person for individualized interventions with a rehabilitation professional.

- If pain is a problem, see Pain CAP.

- If balance is a problem, see Falls CAP.

- If sufficient food intake is a problem, see Undernutrition CAP.

- Refer to self-management programs those persons who have chronic conditions that may fluctuate in intensity or predispose them to flare-ups or acute events. The more confidence the person has in managing his or her health condition, the greater the potential for adherence to an exercise program.

- It is important to recognize that modest increases in activity levels may have beneficial effects. Training programs that are too strenuous are unlikely to be followed and may pose immediate risks to the health of the person.

Provide feedback and rewards if possible.

- Develop a written set of goals and time lines so that the person, family, and formal staff can chart progress and recognize when key milestones have been reached.

- Be prepared to give feedback to the person and family in multiple outcome areas including balance, absence of falls, mobility, endurance, pain, mood, and specific goal attainment.

Additional Resources

Heyn P. 2003. The effect of a multisensory exercise program on engagement, behavior, and selected physiological indexes in persons with dementia. *American Journal of Alzheimer's Disease and Other Dementias* (18,4): 247–51.

Holmberg SK. 1997. A walking program for wanderers: Volunteer training and development of an evening walker's group. *Geriatric Nursing* (18,4): 160–65.

MacRae PG, Asplund LA, Schnelle JF, Ouslander JG, Abrahamse A, Morris C. 1996. A walking program for nursing home residents: Effects on walk endurance, physical activity, mobility, and quality of life. *JAGS* (44,2): 175–80.

Martin JL, Marler MR, Harker JO, Josephson KR, Alessi CA. 2007. A multicomponent nonpharmacological intervention improves activity rhythms among nursing home residents with disrupted sleep/wake patterns. *The Journals of Gerontology Series A: Biological Sciences and Medical Sciences* 62: 67–72.

Miriam Hospital Physical Activity Research Center: www.lifespan.org/behavmed/researchphysical.htm

Nelson ME, Rejeski WJ, Blair SN, Dubcan PW, et al. 2007. Physical activity and public health in older adults. Recommendations from the American College of Sports Medicine and the American Heart Association. *Circulation*: 116.

University of Rhode Island Cancer Prevention Research Center: www.uri.edu/research/cprc/transtheoretical.htm

---

Authors

Katherine Berg, PhD, PT
John N. Morris, PhD, MSW

Instrumental Activities of Daily Living CAP

Problem

This CAP identifies persons who have the capacity and interest to carry out instrumental activities of daily living (IADLs) more independently. The targeted IADLs include preparing meals, doing ordinary housework (washing dishes, making beds, dusting, tidying up, and so on), shopping, and using public transportation or driving oneself. A loss of full self-sufficiency in IADLs is often the first expression of a later, more widespread general decline in functioning. An estimated 17 to 30% of older adults living in the community have IADL problems, with these numbers rising to about 50% of persons living in elderly housing, and over 95% of persons receiving home care. Of persons who are independent in almost all ADLs but who require assistance in the early-loss ADL of bathing, almost all (about 98%) will also have an IADL problem.

For persons with both interest and capacity to carry out IADLs more independently, there is high potential for useful interventions.

Overall Goals of Care

- Preserve current IADL self-sufficiency levels for as long as possible and improve performance if functioning is below capacity.

- Monitor for recent acute events, chronic conditions, or symptoms (such as pain) that influence functional status.

- Review and monitor medications.

- Evaluate effect of motivation and mood on functional status.

- Counsel persons on importance of physical activity and exercise, and provide self-management education.

- Depending on level of function, refer persons who are performing below capacity, and especially those who have recently worsened (for example, in the past 3 months), to community programs, exercise counseling, or specialized physical therapy (PT) or occupational therapy (OT) services.

- Discuss preferences for alternate living arrangements for those who have no interest in continuing or assuming responsibility for IADLs

---

IADL CAP Trigger

This CAP applies to persons living in home care, assisted living, and independent community housing. Its goal is to identify a subset of persons who are capable of and interested in improving their ability to perform these activities. Four key observations are used to identify persons who will trigger this CAP. First, there must be a belief that the person could improve (including those who have recently declined in functioning). This belief can also be considered a proxy for motivation. Second, the person must have at least some moderate dependency in performing IADLs. Third, the person must not be fully dependent in more basic functioning, as represented by Activities of Daily Living (ADLs) such as dressing. Finally, the person must have at least some cognitive capabilities.

TRIGGERED WITH POTENTIAL TO IMPROVE

This group includes persons who display all four of the following key characteristics:

- **Could improve** — Presence of one or more of the following four items:

    - Person believes she or he could be more independent,

    - Assessor believes person could be more independent,

    - Person judged to have good prospects of recovering from current disease [**Note:** Not an item in interRAI's integrated suite but in version 2.0], and

    - ADL status has become worse.

- **IADL difficulty (capacity)** — A total of 3 or higher (or 7 or higher on interRAI's new suite) on the scale produced by summing the codes for the following difficulty/capacity items: meal preparation, ordinary housework, shopping, and transportation.

- **ADL performance** — A score of 0, 1, 2, or 3 on the ADL Hierarchy Scale, representing levels from "independent" to "receiving extensive assistance with early-loss ADLs."

- **Cognitive performance** — A score of 0, 1, or 2 on the Cognitive Performance Scale (levels from "independent" to "mild impairment").

This triggered group includes 20% of persons receiving home care and 2% of older adults living independently in the community. Over a 90-day period, 15% of this group in a home care program will become more independent in IADL performance. The goal is to increase this percentage.

NOT TRIGGERED

This group includes all other persons. This accounts for about 80% of persons receiving home care and 98% of older adults living independently in the community. For those in this group with IADL deficits, an appropriate response would be limited to providing services that complement the care provided by family and friends.

IADL CAP Guidelines

The following guidelines apply to those persons who trigger the IADL CAP, because they should have the capacity for increased independence in IADLs.

Approach to improve IADL performance:

- Speak with the person and family to identify recent changes. Newly occurring medical issues, pharmacological changes, or recurrence of chronic problems can result in functional decline. Note whether IADL performance is now worse than before the precipitating event. If so, improvement can be expected following resolution of the acute problem, while further decline can be expected if the evolving problem is not addressed.

■ Implement monitoring.

Monitor for an acute health problem or the flare-up of a recurrent or chronic problem. Pay particular attention to recent falls, pain, mood, infections, delirium, medications, undernutrition, and vision problems.

■ **Falls** — A history of falls usually triggers a program to address issues of balance, postural dizziness, muscle strength, reduced stamina, overly cautious movements, and loss of range of motion (for example, bending, reaching). Thus, if the Falls CAP is triggered, look for the possibility of benefits as the person improves in these areas. [See Falls CAP.]

■ **Pain** — One-third to one-half of older adults living independently in the community will experience pain, and the resultant course of care begun when the Pain CAP is triggered will often lead to a decrease of pain levels. Thus, if the Pain CAP is triggered, look for improvement in IADLs as pain is managed. [See Pain CAP.]

■ **Mood** — Depression can affect IADL performance because of both withdrawal from activities and the fatigue often associated with this condition. [See Mood CAP.] However, also recognize that the reverse can happen: Decreased IADL capability can result in increased mood problems or decreased feelings of well-being. Thus, improvements in IADLs may have a positive effect on mood state.

■ **Infection or other acute events** can affect IADL performance due to secondary effects of inactivity and fatigue.

■ **Delirium** can affect IADL performance because of an inability to accomplish usual daily tasks. [See Delirium CAP.]

■ **Medications** — Drugs such as anxiolytics, antipsychotics, antidepressants, and hypnotics may induce side effects that result in IADL decline. Consider other drugs that can produce dizziness, hypotension, syncope, balance problems, gait disturbance, and falls. Medication noncompliance or discontinued medication may also contribute to IADL decline. Review the results of the Medications CAP to determine whether medications are contributing to the IADL problem.

■ **Monitor nutrition status** if there has been recent weight loss or a low Body Mass Index. [See Undernutrition CAP.]

■ **Vision** problems and deteriorating vision can have profound effects on IADL tasks. Rehabilitation strategies and technical aids are available to improve performance in IADLs despite vision loss.

Identify strengths. Persons with good cognition and especially strong motivation will be most able to develop and maintain a program to address IADL loss. Those persons with sufficient financial resources will have greater options to purchase PT and OT services, join an exercise program, or purchase an assistive device. The availability of supportive family or friends will also help the person through encouragement, co-participation, and assistance.

Address functional problems. About one-half of the observed improvements in IADLs will occur as persons experience improvements in more basic ADL function, cognition, and communication. [See ADL CAP, Cognition Loss CAP, and Communication CAP.] The CAPs in these three areas provide useful information for improving the person's performance. The key from an IADL perspective is to make a conscious link between improvements in these three areas and potential improvements in IADLs. For example, as you note an improvement in ADLs, ask whether this opens opportunities for the person to become more self-sufficient in IADL activities. In fact, assume the answer is "yes." Give the person the opportunity to become more involved in the basic IADLs, for example, helping to assemble the ingredients to cook a meal, mixing the ingredients, or setting the table.

Often, the ADL plan of care will be the primary strategy for introducing a program that will lead to IADL improvements. If the underlying limitation lies in physical performance, review the ADL and Falls CAPs for suggestions to improve balance, strength, and endurance. Depending on the person's level of functioning, exercise programs may be done alone at home, in community centers, or in clubs; alternately, addressing these problems may require a formal specialized program by a physical therapist.

- **Assess the person's detailed performance and opportunities for increased involvement in IADL.** If a person has difficulty with an IADL, break it down into a series of subtasks. For example, meal preparation can be broken down into retrieving food from storage, preparing each item, combining them as needed, cooking them, and serving the meal. Involvement may be encouraged at different steps until the person becomes more confident in performance. Difficulties should be examined to determine whether the underlying problems reflect strength, balance, coordination, or cognitive or organizational problems. From this analysis, seek to identify the specific action or part of an IADL activity for which an assistive device or environmental modification is needed, where skills retraining may be helpful [see ADL CAP], or where the person could be involved if given the opportunity. An occupational therapist may be helpful in both analyzing and making appropriate recommendations.

- **Assess the person's knowledge and skills.** Sometimes, an IADL problem is associated with a lack of skills or knowledge about performance of tasks previously performed by others, such as a spouse. This is relevant to widowed or divorced men when required to do housekeeping, cooking, and shopping — tasks they may have seldom or never before performed. The same may be true for older women with yard work or managing money (paying bills, balancing a checkbook). In these circumstances, the assessment should focus on both the person's willingness and ability to learn new skills to achieve greater IADL independence. Assume the ability is there and schedule practice sessions. For example, take the person on a supermarket outing or sit with the person as he or she writes and posts checks.

- **It is also important to improve knowledge and skills in self-management of chronic conditions.** These are particularly important for conditions that may have flare-ups or reoccur. Check for local availability of self-management programs.

- **Seek opportunities for increased self-performance of IADLs.** Informal caregivers often assume responsibility for IADL activities which, if given sufficient time, the person could either perform or at least assist in performing. It is important that persons be allowed to function within their capacity, and even to expand on their capacity as they display an ability to carry out IADL tasks. Build on a person's strengths.

- **Motivation.** Motivation is a key strength. Persons who are motivated and believe that they have the potential to improve are more likely to demonstrate improvement in performance. Persons with better cognitive function may also be easier to engage in activity programs. Not all persons are motivated to maintain their past level of involvement in IADLs. They may have extended themselves in the past to perform these activities and now, tired, they are seeking help with them. It is important to assess IADL status even for persons known to be receiving help. It is not uncommon for persons to report the need for more help than they are receiving. Some will need training or services, while others may need only counseling and reassurance. Family or friends may assist with IADLs or provide companionship and assurances. However, it is important to avoid premature substitution, that is, the taking over of IADL tasks in which the person was involved previously. "Doing for the person" is often a poor approach to care. Family education on the benefits of active participation is important.

Cognitive training programs. Formal programs that assist with reasoning, decision making, memory, and visual processing have demonstrated effectiveness in reducing functional decline in IADL performance. [See Cognitive Loss CAP.]

Preference alternatives. If a person is no longer interested in assuming responsibility for IADLs or has never been interested, explore alternatives. This situation may arise following the death of a spouse who previously did all the cooking, cleaning, or yard work.

- Begin counseling on the importance of physical activity and exercise, particularly if the person is no longer performing IADLS or has had a decline in activity. [See Physical Activities Promotion CAP.]

- Explore alternate resources for either informal assistance or paid help.

- Initiate discussion on moving to alternate locations such as a continuing care retirement community, a seniors' residence, or an assisted living setting that provides services for meal preparation and housework.

- If considering a move, suggest questions that should be asked of each potential alternative location. For example, check the type and availability of different activities and exercise programs such as strengthening equipment, dance classes, aquatics, and walking groups. Ideally, look for the availability of activities that the person has enjoyed in the past, enjoys now, or is interested in trying.

- Counsel persons to engage in activities that stimulate cognitive function such as bridge, chess, and puzzles. These skills assist in maintenance of IADLs such as finance and medication management.

- Refer persons to self-management programs for their chronic conditions, so that they are better prepared to adjust to fluctuations in status and recover from flare-ups or other acute problems.

Additional Resources

Elzen H, Slaets JP, Snijders TA, Steverink N. 2007. Evaluation of the chronic disease self-management program (CDSMP) among chronically ill older people in the Netherlands. *Soc Sci Med.* 64(9): 1832–41. Epub 2007, March 13.

Fujita K, Fujiwara Y, Chaves PH, Motohashi Y, Shinkai S. 2006. Frequency of going outdoors as a good predictor for incident disability of physical function as well as disability recovery in community-dwelling older adults in rural Japan. *J Epidemiology* 16(6): 261–70.

Graff MJL, Vernooij-Dassen MJM, Thijssen M, Decker J, Hoefnagels WHL, Rikkert MGMO. 2006. Community based occupational therapy for patients with dementia and their caregivers: Randomized controlled trial. *BMJ* 333: 1196.

Tinetti ME, Allore H, Araujo KL, Seeman T. 2005. Modifiable impairments predict progressive disability among older persons. *Journal of Aging Health* 17(2): 239–56.

Williams CS, Tinetti ME, Kasl SV, Peduzzi PN. 2006. The role of pain in the recovery of instrumental and social functioning after hip fracture. *Journal of Aging Health* 18(5): 743–62.

Willis SL, Tennstedt SL, Marsiske M, Ball K, Elias J, Koepke KM, Morris JN, Rebok GW, Unverzagt FW, Stoddard AM, Wright E. 2006. ACTIVE study group: Long-term effects of cognitive training on everyday functional outcomes in older adults. *JAMA* 296(23): 2805–14.

Authors

John N. Morris, PhD, MSW
Katherine Berg, PhD, PT
Catherine Hawes, PhD
Brant E. Fries, PhD

Activities of Daily Living CAP

Problem

The Activities of Daily Living CAP addresses the person's self-sufficiency in performing basic tasks of daily living, including dressing, personal hygiene, walking, transferring, toileting, changing position in bed, and eating.

A decline in a person's ADL self-sufficiency can lead to a wide variety of complications. These complications can include an increase in incontinence, poor communication, cognitive loss, social isolation, depression, falls, and pressure ulcers. For those living in the community, a decline in ADL self-sufficiency is a major precipitator of the person being transferred to a more supervised setting (for example, moving in with others or being transferred to an assisted living or long-term care setting) and can lead to increased use of formal support services.

Many conditions can affect a person's ADL independence. Among the more important include a decline in cognitive performance, the onset or flare-up of a recurrent chronic disease (for example, depression), the emergence of an acute disease (for example, stroke) or health problem (for example, hip fracture), and the inappropriate use of medications.

While new conditions of this type (and especially advancing dementia) can lead to chronic loss of independence in ADLs, following a plan that encourages ADL self-performance often can slow or even reverse functional decline.

Overall Goals of Care

- Preserve current ADL self-sufficiency levels for as long as possible.

- Monitor a list of specific, potentially troubling acute problems or conditions that can be improved.

- Reverse functional loss resulting from a recent acute event or a condition that can be improved.

- Prevent further functional loss associated with new acute events or a flare-up of chronic conditions that can be improved.

- Improve performance if functioning below capacity.

- Target specific ADL task(s), based on identified inconsistencies between capacity and self-performance, and carry out interventions to improve individualized ADLs.

- Consider referral for physiotherapy (PT) or occupational therapy (OT) services for persons whose ADL function is worse now than 3 months ago or who are performing below capacity.

The goal of this CAP is to improve performance or prevent avoidable functional decline in persons who already have some ADL deficits. The CAP applies to persons living in independent community housing, persons receiving services from home care programs, persons in assisted living housing, and persons residing in nursing homes (long-stay care residents). The following rules specify the two types of persons triggered for specialized follow-up. A key difference between the two triggered groups is whether the person has a fluctuating functional status or condition at the initial assessment, often indicative of a person who has had a recent acute event.

TRIGGERED TO FACILITATE IMPROVEMENT

Included in this group are persons who have all the following characteristics:

- Receive at least some help in ADLs (but are not totally dependent in all ADLs).
- Have at least some minimal cognitive assets (as indicated by having a Cognitive Performance Scale [CPS] score of less than 6).
- Are not at imminent risk of dying.
- And, have two or more of the following indicators that suggest the person has experienced a recent acute event or has a fluctuating functional status:
  - Experiencing an acute episode or a flare-up of a chronic condition
  - Delirium
  - Changing cognitive status (either improving or worsening)
  - Pneumonia
  - Fall
  - Hip fracture
  - Receiving physical therapy
  - Recent hospitalization
  - Fluctuating ADLs (either improving or deteriorating)
  - Fluctuating care needs (with service supports either increasing or decreasing)

This group includes about 20% of persons in long-term care facilities, 20% of persons receiving home care, and less than 1% of older adults living independently in the community. In a long-term care facility setting, about 33% of the persons triggered into this group will improve over a 90-day period; the rate of improvement in home care is about 21%. At the same time, however, this group is in a precarious position. In long-term care facilities, about 33% will decline over the ensuing 90-day period, while in home care the 90-day decline rate is about 20%.

Principal Approach to Care

Manage the new onset acute problem and work to return the person to his or her pre-acute functional level. Second, watch to ensure the person does not enter a cycle of spiraling ADL decline. About 70% of persons experiencing these types of acute health problems will have either recently declined in ADLs or are at elevated risk of decline over the following 90-day period. For a person who experienced a decline in ADLs at the time of the acute health event, addressing the acute health problem is a key step to the person's return to his or her pre-event functional status.

As the acute problem is relieved, work to make sure the functional loss is reversed to the maximum extent possible.

Also recognize that not all acute-related ADL decline is avoidable. Even with excellent ADL self-maintenance programs, up to 20% of persons with recent onset acute health events will experience a decline in ADL. However, in all cases, reversal of the acute health event and recovery of ADL status is a reasonable goal of care.

TRIGGERED TO PREVENT DECLINE

Included in this group are persons who have all the following characteristics:

- Receive at least some help in ADLs (but are not totally dependent in all ADLs).

- Have at least some minimal level of cognitive assets (as indicated by having a Cognitive Performance Scale score of less than 6).

- Are not at imminent risk of dying.

- And, have **none or only one** of the indicators listed under "Triggered to facilitate improvement." This suggests the person has experienced no more than one recent acute event and does not manifest a fluctuating functional status.

This group includes about 60% of persons in long-term care facilities, 15% of persons receiving home care, and less than 1% of older adults living independently in the community. In a long-term care facility setting, about 33% of the persons triggered into this group will improve over a 90-day period, while 32% will decline. The rate of improvement in home care is about 12%, while the decline rate is about 20%.

Principal Approach to Care

The following two-step strategy is recommended:

- Institute a plan of care to help the person preserve current ADL self-sufficiency levels.

- Watch for the onset of acute health problems or new medications that could drive ADL decline (for example, delirium, change in cognition, pneumonia, new hospitalization) and treat or respond in the earliest phase. The onset of such acute problems will be the principal force that drives functional decline in the months ahead.

NOT TRIGGERED

Included in this group is anyone for whom neither functional recovery nor maintenance to prevent functional decline is the overall goal of care. This group is made up of **three distinct subgroups of persons**:

- The first comprises those persons who independently perform even such early-loss ADLs as dressing and personal hygiene (includes most of the persons receiving home care or living independently in the community who are not triggered).

- The second comprises those who have no residual functional or cognitive assets (CPS score of 6).

- The third comprises those persons who are at imminent risk of dying.

The two latter subgroups make up most of those in long-term care facilities who are not triggered on this CAP.

This group includes about 20% of persons in long-term care facilities, 65% of persons receiving home care, and 99% of older adults living independently in the community. In a long-term care facility setting, about 25% of the persons triggered into this group will decline over a 90-day period, while 12% will improve. The equivalent rate of improvement in home care is about 14%, while the decline rate is about 14%.

- Appropriate ADL monitoring and maintenance care are warranted for those persons with ADL deficits for whom functional recovery or maintenance may not be possible.

Activities of Daily Living CAP Guidelines

Most service programs successfully reach out to some of the persons identified by the ADL CAP triggers, but miss others and provide care to those who would not benefit. Through this ADL review, a greater number of appropriate persons for ADL improvement or maintenance care will be reached and needless functional decline avoided. This approach targets those persons who will benefit most from intensive assessment, monitoring, and intervention. The care can be reasonably performed in any program setting. Care plans and ongoing monitoring will provide extensive interventions to some and less to others.

Approach to improve ADL performance:

- Speak with the person, family, and caregivers to identify new acute episodes. Newly occurring medical, pharmacologic, orthopedic, or vision problems can result in precipitous rates of functional decline. When such conditions occur, note whether ADL functional decline follows. If so, improvement can be expected following the resolution of the acute problem; if ADL issues are not addressed, further decline can be expected. Thus, a referral to a physician is recommended, with information provided on noted clinical changes and consequent functional decline.

- Implement a monitoring program to

    - Inform family and caregivers of the need to watch for the onset of major acute problems that could lead to functional decline (for example, delirium, pneumonia, falls, and hip fractures). When observed, refer the person to a physician.

    - Inform family and caregivers of the need to detect evolving chronic conditions that could lead to functional decline, and especially those that are remediable, such as cataracts or osteoarthritis of the hip or knee.

    - Monitor for inappropriate use of medications leading to functional decline (a newly administered medication, but also a discontinued drug).

    - Check for ADL decline or a drop in activity levels following a recent return from the hospital.

- If symptoms of delirium are present, deliver care in line with the Delirium CAP guidelines. As a part of this effort, review medications to identify drugs that may contribute to delirium and interfere with functioning.

- If dizziness, falls, or recent hip fracture are present, see Falls CAP.

- If the person recently declined or is performing below capacity, refer to or consult with PT or OT, if possible. Persons in this category who receive PT and OT have almost double the rate of improvement over a 90-day period as compared to similar persons who do not receive such care.

- Physicians and other members of the interdisciplinary team need to assess and treat the underlying medical problems.

- If indicators of inadequate nutritional status are present, implement nutritional intervention. [See Undernutrition CAP.]

- If indicators of inadequate pain management are present, review management strategies. [See Pain CAP.]

Review the two interRAI assessment items on the staff's and the person's views of whether further improvements in function are possible. Improvements in performance are more likely and less ADL decline is expected if the person and the staff believe improvement is possible. These items should help guide your view of how to plan and carry out care and services for the person.

Address chronic cognitive loss. Cognitive loss affects a person's potential for ADL improvement and makes it more difficult to lessen functional decline. The cognitive performance items from the interRAI assessment are useful in assessing a person's functional capacity and potential for ADL improvement. Specifically, several of the items in the Cognitive Performance Scale (CPS) can help guide your thinking even when the CPS itself is not calculated. These items include short term memory, decision making, and ability to be understood. [**Note:** See scoring of key interRAI scales for specific guidance on the CPS. The CPS score should be available in your software system.]

- Persons with the greatest deficit in cognition (those with a CPS score of 6) are not triggered on this CAP, as their lack of mental capabilities provide only minimal capacity to improve.

- All other persons are triggered, as ADL performance can often be improved or at least preserved in persons with a CPS score of less than 6.

- Those with no impairment or even persons with moderately impaired cognition (CPS scores of 0, 1, and 2) have the best capacity to improve in ADL.

- Persons with moderately to severely impaired cognition (CPS scores of 3, 4, and 5) need a highly structured ADL plan of care.

Select targeted ADLs for care interventions to prevent further decline and increase independence by comparing self-performance vs. capacity. ADL loss follows a regular, hierarchical pattern. Typically, persons first need help with the so-called "early-loss" ADLs (bathing, dressing, and personal hygiene), followed by the need for help with "middle-loss" ADLs (walking, transfer, toileting), and finally help with "late-loss" ADLs (eating and bed mobility).

- To help preserve — or even improve — ADL self-performance, the person, family, and caregivers can target a specific ADL area for review and potential improvement. For example:

  - For those who are fully independent in walking, focus on an "early-loss" ADL (usually dressing).

  - Focus on "walking" for someone who still has some ability to walk, but is not totally independent.

  - For those who are dependent in walking, focus the care plan on a "late-loss" ADL (usually eating). For example, if the person can still ingest solid foods, provide opportunity and encouragement to self feed. If triggered on the Undernutrition CAP, follow those instructions for such a person.

- Having selected the ADL area around which a program to increase independence will be based, there are many ways to develop a suitable approach to facilitate improvement.

  - At the more formal end of the spectrum of possible approaches, referrals to therapists or an in-house exercise program may be choices often considered. Also consider building a situation-based ADL maintenance and rehabilitation program, focusing on the targeted ADL area. Such an approach is described in the following section.

- At the less formal end of the spectrum of possible approaches, the person and a key family member can be educated on how to facilitate this type of program. Begin by explaining that increased independence is possible. Setting an appropriate expectation is key to change. Then suggest that the person follow a personal version of the formal program described below. The critical elements are as follows: pick an ADL subtask on which to seek greater independence, provide an opportunity for the person to do the subtask, keep track of success and failure, and build upon instances of success.

Example approach to situation-based ADL maintenance and rehabilitation:

- Provide verbal instructions or cueing for each step of a targeted program addressing a specific ADL function.

- Give the person the opportunity to start the activity step, helping as needed.

- Use gestures or verbal cues to which the person responds.

- When a person needs help with a selected task, break the task into segments and set goals for improvement within both tasks and segments.

- Have all care professionals and family members use the same approach every time the ADL activity is performed.

- Continue to use this consistent approach for at least 1 month.

- Document progress in how the person engages in the selected ADL task and each task segment. Note changes in how the person begins the task, if cueing or assistance is needed to start, and if he or she can manage to complete the task once started. It may also be useful in measuring progress to document the time required to complete each task or subtask.

- Share improvements with caregivers, the person, and family. Sometimes small improvements may not be noticeable to everyone. When well documented, they can be encouraging to everyone involved.

Consequence of functional loss of ADL. Functional loss can also lead to the onset of new problems, including, for example, incontinence, social isolation, depression, falls, accidents, and pressure ulcers. Look for the new onset of such conditions and, as ADLs improve, look for corresponding improvements in these areas.

Authors

John N. Morris, PhD, MSW
Katherine Berg, PhD, PT
Jean-Claude Henrard, MD
Harriet Finne-Soveri, MD, PhD
Dinnus Frijters, PhD

Home Environment Optimization CAP

Problem

The Home Environment Optimization CAP focuses on the home environment, looking at features generally classified as environmental hazards. These include such items as general disrepair, poor lighting, unsafe flooring and rugs, inadequate heating or cooling, faulty appliances, and a general state of squalor. The focus of this review is broad and addresses concerns with life safety, falls, health status, and basic quality of life.

Resolving these problems is often a challenge. The person living on a modest income may have made decisions that contributed to the situation (for example, paying for food rather than heat). Such a person may have little personal physical or financial reserves to address these problems. Available public support programs or services may have limited funds to correct environmental deficits, or their program entitlement guidelines may restrict who can be helped and how funds can be expended. Finally, alternative housing may be in limited supply, with a long waiting list and restricted eligibility, while family may be unable to provide an alternative setting for the person.

At a minimum, this environmental assessment identifies hazards that can be corrected relatively easily. For a more successful implementation of a residential improvement program, the person and his or her key informal caregiver should be included in the decision-making process. For some, acceptance of recommended changes is a process that occurs over time. It is important for the assessor to understand the person's resistance to change, including feelings of potential loss, shame, or inadequacy, as well as denial of the problem.

Overall Goal of Care

- Improve the safety of the environment in which the person lives.

Home Environment Optimization CAP Trigger

This CAP triggers for frail adults who live in the community in a home environment with problematic features and who have physical or mental conditions that complicate these problems or allow the problems to put the person at higher risk of adverse outcomes.

TRIGGERED

Persons who exhibit **both** of the following conditions:
- The home environment has **one or more** of the following:
    - Lighting problem
    - Flooring or carpeting problem
    - Bathroom or toilet problem

- Kitchen problem
- Heating or cooling problem
- Significant disrepair of the home
- Squalid conditions

- The person has **two or more** of the following indicators of frailty:
  - Not able to climb stairs
  - Less than 2 hours of physical activity in the last 3 days
  - Unsteady gait
  - Poor health
  - Conditions or diseases that make the person unstable
  - Difficult access to the home
  - Difficult access to rooms in the home
  - Depression Rating Scale (DRS) of 3 or higher
  - Any one of three mental-health symptoms: hallucinations, delusions, abnormal thoughts

This triggered group includes about 15% of persons receiving home care and 2% of adults living independently in the community. Of those triggered, about one-half will have problems with flooring and bathrooms, while one-quarter or less will have problems in the other areas.

NOT TRIGGERED   Includes all other persons. This group includes about 85% of persons receiving home care.

Home Environment Optimization CAP Guidelines

Not all of the environmental conditions covered in this CAP will require immediate intervention. Although some conditions represent clear hazards (for example, an absence of heat in cold weather), others may represent only a slight hazard or may have only a minimal impact on the person's function (for example, high doorsills for those who are restricted to wheelchairs or a squalid condition with excessive hoarding). Given these thoughts, the following approaches are relevant.

Heating and cooling. A failure to maintain an appropriate temperature in the home can place the person at risk of hypothermia or hyperthermia. When this risk is present, immediate action is needed to correct the problem.

- Does the person's medical condition or degree of frailty prohibit him or her from sensing the temperature in the home?

- Does the person suffer from a condition that is likely to prevent him or her from performing a basic activity such as setting the thermostat: depression (for example, a DRS score of 3 or higher), severe malnourishment (triggered by the Undernutrition CAP), or excessive daily consumption of alcohol? [See Tobacco and Alcohol Use CAP.]

- Is the problem made worse by economic issues? If yes, is there a solution?
  - Does the community have fuel assistance, weatherization, or home modification programs for low-income homeowners and renters?

- Is there a relative who could help the person in either managing the heating/cooling or in providing economic assistance with home utilities?

- Is the person making poor choices (such as spending money on alcohol) or is he or she generally unable to manage his or her own finances? The caregiver, relatives, or friends may be able to provide advice or assistance in designing a more appropriate budget.

Lighting. Simple corrective steps are often all that will be needed, including replacing burned-out bulbs, increasing bulb wattage, installing night-lights, or providing more lamps.

Flooring and carpeting. Some easy strategies to be considered include

- Avoid scatter rugs.

- Adhere rugs to the floor using double-sided tape.

- Use a bath mat with nonskid backing.

- Repair loose flooring and holes in the floor or carpet. If the person does not have the money to make repairs, identify others who could help (for example, a volunteer group in the community, a relative, or a church member).

- For persons with mobility problems, home modifications including space, width of doorways and hallways, doorsills, ramps, and other safety installations may be warranted.

General space requirements. Mobility aids such as wheelchairs and walkers require a significant amount of space within rooms, corridors, and bathrooms to permit independent use. For instance, wheelchairs require a turning radius of 5 feet and wider doorways. Removal of doorsills or doors may be warranted, and furniture and room contents may need to be rearranged or removed. Absence of such accommodations is to blame for higher rates of injuries among wheelchair users.

Bathroom. About one-half of all serious falls occur in the bathroom. If possible, properly installed permanent hand supports and grab bars should be present, although arranging for installation of such support devices can be difficult. As a first step, identify any community groups that may be willing to help. Also speak with the person and family about their ability to have the support devices installed.

Kitchen. Stove-related fires are a critical risk. Preventive measures include using a timer, having another person cook, or cooking only when someone else is present. For persons who have a history of hazardous use of the stove, consider using childproof knobs, installing a cutoff switch, or shutting down the stove and only using a microwave.

- Make sure smoke alarms and fire extinguishers are present, working, and in a known location. Discuss an emergency plan with the person and family, ensuring there is a common strategy in place (for example, emergency alert call system).

- Check that necessary safety equipment is within reach and that the placement of the stove does not put it at risk of igniting flammable materials such as curtains or of having something fall on the stove, thereby causing a fire. Consider alterations in layout of the kitchen or need for structural modification.

- Alternative housing may be necessary if the person lives alone or if it is not possible to make necessary modifications to the home.

State of disrepair of the home or squalid conditions. Look for general clutter as well as frayed wiring, overloaded electrical circuits, broken stairs, shattered windows, leaky pipes, rat and bug infestation, clogged drains or toilets, pet feces, and old garbage. First try to identify why these conditions exist (for example, cognitive or functional impairment, absence of money, lack of any other place to live) and then offer possible remedial steps.

If self-neglect due to depression or mental health issues is the key barrier, notify the person's physician and consider referral for a mental health assessment.

Neighborhood. Assessment of safety of the community or neighborhood.

Additional Resources

AARP Home Design. www.aarp.org/families/home_design/

Berg K, Hines M, Allen SM. 2002. Wheelchair users at home: Few home modifications and many injurious falls. *American Journal of Public Health* 92: 48.

Gitlin LN, Winter L, Dennis MP, Corcoran M, Schinfeld S, Hauck WW. 2006. A randomized trial of a multicomponent home intervention to reduce functional difficulties in older adults. *JAGS* (May) 54(5): 809–16.

Misset B, De Jonghe B, Bastuji-Garin S, Gattolliat O, Boughrara E, Annane D, Hausfater P, Garrouste-Orgeas M, Carlet J. 2006. Mortality of patients with heatstroke admitted to intensive care units during the 2003 heat wave in France: A national multiple-center risk-factor study. *Critical Care Medicine* (April) 34(4): 1087–92.

Van Bemmel T, Vandenbroucke JP, Westendorp RG, Gussekloo J. 2005. In an observational study elderly patients had an increased risk of falling due to home hazards. *Journal of Clinical Epidemiology* (January) 58(1): 63–67.

Authors

Catherine Hawes, PhD
Brant E. Fries, PhD
Dinnus Frijters, PhD
Knight Steel, MD
Rosemary Bakker, MS
John N. Morris, PhD, MSW
Katherine Berg, PhD, PT

Section 5

Institutional Risk CAP

Problem

The Institutional Risk CAP identifies persons who have an increased risk of entering a long-term care facility in the coming months. They typically have deficits in physical functioning, memory, decision making, and health. This CAP describes steps to be taken to lessen the likelihood of entering such a facility.

Most persons identified for this CAP will remain in the community, receiving informal support mainly from family members and modest supplemental support by formal agencies. However, as the person's problems increase in complexity, so too does the likelihood of entering a long-term care facility.

Institutional placement is most likely to occur following a long process of decline. Functional decline typically begins with minor decrements in performing instrumental ADLs (for example, cleaning the home or shopping for groceries). Sensing that something is amiss, family and close friends step forward to help compensate for this new loss. This level of assistance may remain the same for a long period of time, as functional decline is often a remarkably slow process. With time, a person may experience additional problems in day-to-day decision making and memory, and eventually develop dependency in one or more basic ADLs. As the person and others note the loss, informal help increases. The first ADL tasks to require assistance are usually personal hygiene and dressing. The onset of behavioral problems may further complicate the situation.

Although the person and family are usually able to adapt and adjust levels of assistance according to changes in capacity, the person's needs may eventually exceed the capacity of the informal network to provide appropriate support. At this point, the person or key family members believe that entry into a long-term care facility may be in the person's best interests. This may happen after a hospitalization for an acute problem or the flare-up of a recurrent chronic condition. The precipitating event may be a fall, a fracture, pneumonia, or other reason for a prolonged period of inactivity or bed rest. Regardless of the underlying cause, with functional independence further compromised, the person, family, and discharge personnel may consider a long-term care facility admission. However, for many of these persons, institutional admission will often be avoided with appropriate interventions and community supports.

Overall Goal of Care

- Avoid premature admission to a long-term care facility by supporting family efforts and providing community intervention programs.

Institutional Risk CAP Trigger

This CAP trigger identifies persons with impaired functioning who are at high risk of institutional placement in the coming months.

TRIGGERED

This group includes persons who have four or more of following conditions:

- Any stay in a long-term care facility in the past 5 years
- Short-term memory problems
- Any deficit in cognitive skills for daily decision making
- Alzheimer's disease
- Any limitation in making oneself understood
- Any limitation in understanding others
- Any of the following behavioral problems (at any frequency): wandering, verbally abusive, physically abusive, socially inappropriate behavior, inappropriate public sexual behavior, or resists care
- Receiving any help in transfer (or did not occur)
- Receiving any help in locomotion (or did not occur)
- Receiving any help in personal hygiene (or did not occur)
- Decline in ADLs in the prior 90 days
- Wheeled by others (indoors)
- Does not go out of the house
- One or more falls in the last 90 days
- Occasional, frequent, or daily urinary incontinence

This triggered group includes 40% of persons receiving home care and 1% of older adults living independently in the community. About 80% of persons newly admitted for long-stay care in long-term care facilities will meet this trigger condition. For triggered persons in home care, about 20% will enter a long-term care facility within a year — twice the rate of those not triggered. For triggered older adults living independently in the community, about 30% will enter a long-term care facility within 1 year — about four times the rate of those not triggered.

NOT TRIGGERED

All other persons. This group accounts for about 60% of persons receiving home care and 88% of older adults living independently in the community.

Institutional Risk CAP Guidelines

Identifying persons and families who appear ready to make the decision to consider a long-term care facility admission. The following approach may be used to redirect premature decisions to enter a long-term care facility.

- For a person in hospital, assess premorbid levels of function and changes in status following the precipitating event. Consider whether there is a reasonable expectation of partial or full recovery. For the vast majority of persons, declines in functional status will be of recent onset and, in the absence of a massive cognitive loss, there is substantial potential for the person to improve and not need institutionalization. For those who were dependent prior to the precipitating event, determine the level of assistance that family or other caregivers were providing on a routine basis.

- If there has been a fall, review the Falls CAP.

- If delirium is present, review the Delirium CAP.

- If the person is depressed, review the Mood CAP.

- If there has been a decline in ADLs, review the ADL CAP.

- If family is distressed and seems not able to continue the informal caregiving, review the Informal Support CAP.

■ For a person in the community who has not had a recent hospital admission:

- Assess whether decline is related to any of the following:

  • Decisions by the family to do more for the person than may be necessary (for example, a family member, concerned for the person's safety, may have begun to do things for the person without being asked, or the family member does not have the patience to wait when the person performs an activity slowly).
  • Recent changes in medications may cause the person to slow down.

- Do not forget to highlight the person's residual strengths. For example, consider his or her capacity to make decisions, ability to walk, positive outlook, love of grandchildren, financial resources, and determination to stay in the community.

- Ask about any rehabilitation intervention to address previous declines. [See ADL CAP.]

Problem solving through other triggered CAPs. For a person considered at high risk of entering a long-term care facility, the goal is to identify those conditions that can be addressed in the community. For someone triggered on this CAP, consider his or her underlying risk of going into a long-term care facility as part of your review of other triggered CAPs. Some of the major CAP problem areas that may be triggered include

■ ADL decline

■ Falls

■ Cognitive decline

■ Delirium

■ Communication decline

■ Urinary incontinence

■ Behavior problems

The primary task is to ensure that institutional risk status is highlighted, in the above areas, in the plan of care. Knowing that a person is at risk of admission to a long-term care facility should help ensure that identified problems are addressed.

Watch for subsequent loss in any of the areas identified in this CAP trigger: ADLs, memory, decision making, communication, falls, behavior, or bladder function.

■ Identify the new problem or worsening status as soon as possible.

■ Seek to identify changes in health status or care patterns that might explain what has happened to the person — a new disease or medication, or a failure to comply with a prescribed course of care.

- Consider strategies and education for self-management or family education about managing chronic conditions.

Role of family. Most persons will have reasonable family networks that naturally step forward to provide support.

- If family members are providing support today, they are likely to continue to perform in this way in the near term at least. As new needs arise, family members often surprise themselves as they step forward to help their loved one. Nonetheless, it is helpful to provide education to the family and person on self-management strategies, lifestyle changes, and coping strategies, as well as information on expected course of recovery or decline over time.

- At the same time, in the rare instance when the person has a poor informal support system, he or she can be expected to receive significantly less help from family and friends. If true today, this will be true tomorrow. Such informal support systems seldom self-correct. In these instances, you should be prepared to arrange for increased levels of formal care.

- Many key informal helpers will lack information both on what types of changes to expect for the person being helped and on how they can best respond over time. Programs of individual and group counseling, as well as the dissemination of information (either on a real-time, hot-line basis or through brochures on key facts), may be helpful.

- Recognize that the person may suggest going to a long-term care facility or assisted living so as "not to be a burden" on family and loved ones. Often it is an incorrect perception by the person that assistance cannot be continued, especially with additional support of formal care services. Discuss these perceptions with the person and his or her informal caregivers.

- Periodically planned respite care, including in-home or day care for a few hours at a time, or institutional respite care for days or weeks, may enable informal caregivers to sustain a support role for longer periods of time.

Temporary services for urgent problems. When families are severely distressed by the person's new problems, refer them to a social worker or other appropriate professional to identify available formal support resources and housing. Respite care or increases of formal services may be important in keeping the family involved in the care of the person. In other instances, the person may require another housing setting on a temporary basis. This can be due to the absence of a caregiver because of illness or job considerations, or because the person's current residence will no longer be available. In such cases, attention should be directed to why such placements are necessary and to helping informal caregivers set sensible expectations about their responsibilities, duties, and preferences once the person returns home.

Specialized assisted living housing alternatives. To the extent that such resources are available in a community, specialized housing options can be considered. Assisted living housing (independent apartments with barrier-free features and access to supportive services) can have a significant effect on reducing the need for institutionalization. For impaired persons, including those with some cognitive loss and mild to moderate functional problems, assisted living options can be arranged where a partnership of formal and informal services help support the person.

Preventive measures that reduce the risk of events that increase disability. There is increasing evidence that lifestyle measures and medical interventions may reduce the subsequent risk of cardiovascular events or the morbidity arising from them, falls, and further functional decline. Actions that prevent such morbidity also often can reduce the likelihood of needing institutionalization.

Additional Resources

Barusha AJ, Pandav R, Shen C, Dodge HH, Ganguli M. 2004. Predictors of nursing facility admission: A 12-year epidemiological study in the United States. *JAGS* 52: 434–39.

Laukkanen P, Leskinen E, Kauppinen M, Sakari-Rantala R, Heikkinen E. 2000. Health and functional capacity as predictors of community dwelling among elderly people. *Journal of Clinical Epidemiology* 53:257–65.

Payette H, Coulombe C, Boutier V, Gray-Donald K. 2000. Nutrition risk factors for institutionalization in a free-living functionally dependent elderly population. *Journal of Clinical Epidemiology* 53: 579–87.

Soto ME, Andrieu S, Gillette-Guyonnet S, Cantet C, Nourhasheni F, Vellas B. 2006. Risk factors for functional decline and institutionalisation among community-dwelling older adults with mild to severe Alzheimer's disease: One year of follow-up. *Age and Ageing* 35(3): 308–10.

Authors

John N. Morris, PhD, MSW
Jean-Claude Henrard, MD
Brant E. Fries, PhD

Physical Restraints CAP

Problem

This CAP identifies persons who are physically restrained. A restraint is any device (for example, a physical or mechanical device, material, or equipment attached or adjacent to the person's body) that the person cannot easily remove and that restricts freedom of movement or normal access to his or her body. What is important is the effect the device has on the person, not the purpose for which the device was placed on the person. This also includes the use of passive restraints such as chairs that prevent rising. The goal of this CAP is to eliminate the use of restraints by employing appropriate measures as necessary according to the person's physical and/or cognitive abilities.

Physical restraints are associated with negative physical and psychosocial outcomes. They are almost never indicated, and at most should be used only as a short-term temporary intervention. If used for any significant period of time, the physical consequences may include loss of muscle mass, contractures, lessened mobility and stamina, impaired balance, skin breakdown, constipation, and incontinence. Further, persons who try to free themselves from restraints may fall and be injured. There is even a high risk of strangulation when certain types of restraints are used.

The psychosocial effects of restraint use may include a feeling of shame, hopelessness, and stigmatization as well as agitation. Behavior disturbances that are sometimes the excuse for restraint use may even be aggravated. It is sometimes suggested that restraints be used because of staffing shortages. However, there is considerable evidence that the use of restraints increases demands on staff because it is necessary to check the person's status more often than usual throughout the day, and there may be a decline in physical and mental health as well.

Overall Goals of Care

- Identify and treat symptoms related to use of physical restraints.

- Identify and carry out alternative care approaches (for example, restorative care, alternative seating/positioning, individualized activities, or constant monitoring by staff/volunteer).

- Evaluate the use of alternative methods and outcomes in an ongoing manner.

Physical Restraints CAP Trigger

This CAP applies to persons in long-term care facilities and post acute care settings. This CAP does not apply to persons in home care or other community settings.

The Physical Restraints CAP identifies two types of persons for follow-up, using interRAI's ADL Self-Performance Hierarchy Scale. Both groups will be restrained in their movement at the time of assessment by devices such as trunk restraints or chairs that prevent rising. The groups differ in their ADL self-performance status: One group is more self-engaged in ADLs, while the other group has little independence in these activities.

TRIGGERED TO REMOVE RESTRAINTS FOR PERSONS WITH THE ABILITY TO PERFORM SOME MIDDLE- OR EARLY-LOSS ADL ACTIVITIES (for example, personal hygiene, dressing, and walking)

Persons in this subgroup tend to be restrained because of concerns about falling, wandering, and behavioral problems (for example, resisting care, physical abuse, or socially inappropriate behavior). About one in five restrained persons will fall into this group. Organizations with effective restraint reduction programs have been able to eliminate restraints in caring for such persons.

This group includes 1% of persons in long-term care facilities and 2% of persons receiving home care.

TRIGGERED TO REMOVE RESTRAINTS FOR PERSONS WITH LITTLE OR NO ABILITY TO PERFORM MIDDLE- OR EARLY-LOSS ADLs

Persons in this subgroup are more likely to have a history of falls and behavioral problems than the subgroup not triggered. About 70% of these persons have severe cognitive loss and a like number are unable to walk or use a wheelchair. About 40% will be unable to sit upright on their own, over one-quarter will have severe problems in seeing or understanding others, and about 15% will be tube fed. With effective restraint reduction programs, few, if any, such persons will require restraints.

This group includes 1 to 6% of persons in long-term care facilities and less than 1% of persons receiving home care.

NOT TRIGGERED

This group includes persons who do not use physical restraints or a chair that prevents rising. In addition, persons with quadriplegia and those who are comatose are not triggered. Their plan of care would call for the use of proper chairs and support apparatuses.

Physical Restraints CAP Guidelines

Initial Considerations Prior to Temporary Use of a Physical Restraint

There are a limited number of situations where a physical restraint may need to be applied on an emergency basis. An example would be to prevent violence to others, harm to self, or a suicide attempt (consult facility psychiatric practice standards for such emergency use), or to allow an essential medical treatment to proceed. As soon as the immediate concern passes, the person must be evaluated for removal of the restraint and referred for care as described below.

When consideration is being given to the use of a physical restraint at other times, first complete a thorough assessment to consider care approaches that do not involve restraint use. The following are examples of issues to consider:

- **Seating** — Does the person need a different type of seat? Often, restraints are misused as positioning devices.

    - Consider an assessment by a therapist to determine the most suitable seating apparatus given the person's physical condition.

    - When a wheelchair is used for transport only, encourage the person to move to other chairs for more permanent seating during the day. This would not necessarily apply to a wheelchair that has been customized for that person (for example, having tilt/recline, custom back). Such a wheelchair is often the most appropriate seating as compared to standard furniture. Provide access to as many types of seating as reasonable for that person to allow for a change in posture and perhaps a different environment.

- **Ambulation, transfers, and positioning** — What is the person's daily routine? This review may point to ways to individualize the current living environment to reduce the risk of falling by providing the person with the necessary help for transfers, ambulation, or position changes before the person would try such moves unassisted. Consider the times of both day and night when interventions other than restraints can reduce the risk of adverse outcomes.

    - Consider the usual time the person gets out of bed, uses the toilet, is involved in activities, eats meals, rests in bed, and sleeps.

    - Are there opportunities for the person to be repositioned without restraints during meals, activities, and at other times?

    - Does the person use suitable adaptive equipment, including canes and walkers, for mobility? Has the person been trained (if appropriate) and monitored on the proper use of the adaptive equipment?

    - Does the person have suitable nonskid, well-fitting footwear?

For persons already in restraints, determine the reason for their use. If, after this review, the decision is made to temporarily continue using a physical restraint, the person's plan of care must identify the following:

- A detailed rationale for use of the restraint.

- The specific time(s) the restraint(s) is (are) to be used and a detailed schedule for checking the status of the person when it is. Such a schedule will specify the frequency of checking by hour and day. For example, one such plan would call for the person to be checked every 15 minutes for the first 2 days and every hour for the following 5 days.

- Monitor the person's physical and emotional response to the restraint (for example, assess for agitation, calling out, pulling at the restraint, tearfulness).

- Determine the presence of the person's consent (or proxy consent if the person is not capable to provide consent) for the restraint use.

- Design a plan outlining steps to eliminate the use of the restraint as soon as possible.

- Establish a target date by which the restraint will be removed. If this date has passed, re-evaluate in detail the need for restraint use and document the reasons it was not removed by the target date.

Considerations Following Application of a Physical Restraint

Is the person restrained because of a history of falling? [Consult the Falls CAP for a more detailed discussion of falls.] If this is the case, there are two main actions: (1) develop a list of the conditions that may place the person at an increased risk of falling; and (2) develop alternative care strategies for each of the applicable conditions identified in the following section. Restraints are never a correct strategy to address these conditions. The following is a list of common conditions that call for nonrestraint solutions.

- High-risk clinical factors suggesting that severe injury might result should a fall occur. Examples include osteoporosis; severe visual impairment; anticoagulation therapy including wafarin, heparin, or aspirin; recent hip fracture; and a recent episode of syncope.

- Functional limitations that suggest a fall would have a higher likelihood of a serious consequence—for example, the presence of a significant limitation in locomotion or transferring. [See the ADL CAP.]

- Would the person benefit from an exercise or rehabilitation program to improve underlying conditions? Examples include strength training to improve muscle tone, aerobic exercise to increase cardiovascular stamina, and gait and balance training to increase steadiness.

Is the person restrained because of a history of wandering behavior? Restraints are rarely indicated for such behavior and even then only for a matter of a few minutes under most circumstances. Many techniques and devices are now available to address this issue. Alert devices can be placed on the person so that a door automatically locks when the person approaches. Identification bracelets, such as Medical Alert, can be placed on the person for prompt identification. Circular paths that do not have an exit outside may allow the person to walk without being able to leave the building. [See the Behavior CAP for more details on how to address the care of such persons.]

- Does the person wander because of an abnormal cognitive state (for example, short-term memory impairment, impaired cognitive skills for decision making, variations in mental function over the course of the day)? Assess and treat reversible cognitive problems. [See Delirium CAP, Cognitive CAP.]

- Is the person able to make him- or herself understood and can he or she understand others? Note clarity of speech and the person's ability to give and to understand directions and conversation. Provide different forms of communication/directions as needed (for example, wall signs that redirect the person). [See Communication CAP.]

- Determine if the person's need to move could be satisfied through purposeful activity, such as participation in a walking program.

- Determine if there are patterns to wandering or behavior disturbances. Consider what is motivating the person. Consider the time of day and build a routine around the need to wander. Consider the person's prior routine to identify possible activities the person might want to pursue.

- Determine if wandering or behavior disturbances may be a side effect of a medication. [See Behavior CAP.]

- Has the person recently moved into the facility? Is the person trying to deal with loss or fear of the unknown? The care approach should include strategies to make the person feel safe, comfortable, and secure in the care environment.

Is the person restrained because of agitated or abusive behaviors? [Consult the Behavior CAP for a more detailed discussion of behavior management.]

- Does the person have a history of a psychiatric diagnosis? Review the person's medication regimen to ensure that correct medications are being used.

- Determine whether the behavior is the result of an unmet need in a non-behavioral area (for example, pain/discomfort, fatigue, hunger, thirst, fear, bowel/bladder need, boredom or overstimulation, need to move around), and design alternative strategies to meet such needs.

- Is the abusive behavior new? Because an acute medical condition can result in delirium or an acute psychotic episode associated with striking behavioral change, immediate referral to a physician is required if this is a consideration. [See Delirium CAP.]

- Identify any precipitating factor(s), remove them from the environment if possible, and adjust care schedules to reflect the person's unique needs. Examples of treatment strategies include

  - Allow the person to decide to get up in the morning or be bathed.

- Redirect the person with calm, simple, clear, and reassuring directions and remove environmental hazards and other persons from the immediate vicinity. Allow the person to safely express his or her emotions.

- Provide one-on-one intervention/supervision, as tolerated by the person. Many persons who are agitated and pacing may be willing to be accompanied by a staff member while verbally releasing their anger and frustration.

- Avoid speaking in loud, forceful, or urgent tones that may further irritate the person. If the person is being physically abusive, move away and allow the person to have space. This will decrease the person's sense of feeling trapped. Remove others from the situation. When it seems safe, approach the person in a calm, reassuring manner.

- Was abusive behavior toward another person provoked or unprovoked? Identification of provoking factors will aid in determining a suitable plan to prevent future abusive behavior toward others. Examples of treatment strategies include the following:

  - If the person wandered into another's room, a harsh response by the occupant may make the wanderer strike out (behavior provoked).

  - If the abuse was not a result of provocation, consider an immediate referral to a physician while beginning immediate steps to maintain safety of staff and other persons.

  - Approach the person in a calm, quiet, soothing manner. A person often mirrors the behavior of those around him or her.

  - Consider the physical environment and decide if overstimulation or understimulation may be factors that affect abusive outbursts. Proper interventions may include, but are not limited to, adjusting awakening and retiring schedules, adapting meal times, providing one-on-one activities and variations in current activity schedules, adjustment of medications, and referral for medical or psychiatric evaluation and intervention.

  - Take steps to improve the continuity of care (for example, use a primary nursing care approach). Is one staff member assigned to the same person over long periods of time to build up an understanding of his or her individual strengths, preferences, needs, and idiosyncrasies? A sense of familiarity with a consistent caregiver may reduce and even eliminate periods of abusive behavior.

Is the person restrained to prevent the removal of an essential medical device (for example, IV tube or tracheostomy tube)?

- What is the person communicating by trying to remove a medical device? Could it be localized pain at a tube insertion site that could be corrected? Did the person express wishes to not have a tube before it was inserted? Is the person trying to convey his or her wishes? Consider discussions with the person, family, and health care team to review the goals of care and the person's wishes about health care treatments.

- Is a family member able to spend time with the person to calm and reassure him or her?

- If a device is considered necessary, interventions to distract the person from pulling at it include the following:

  - Dress the person in a long-sleeved shirt to cover tubing in the arm.

  - Dress the person in long pants with a leg bag to discourage pulling at an indwelling catheter.

- Dress the person in a turtleneck shirt to keep him or her from reaching for a subclavian line.

- Offer the person something to hold to occupy his or her hands (for example, putty, a foam ball, rosary beads, a clean piece of tubing, or a personal possession small enough to hold).

- Invite the person to attend activities that keep the person actively involved.

- Arrange for a sitter or a video monitor.

- If treatment is temporary (for example, IV antibiotics) and the above alternatives do not work, consider the least restrictive form of restraint, closely monitor the person, and devise a plan to remove the restraint as soon as possible.

Additional Resources

"Everyone wins! Quality care without restraints." 1995. The Independent Production Fund, in association with Toby Levine Communications, Inc., New York, NY.

Tideiksaar, R. 1998. Preventing falls, avoiding restraints. *Untie the Elderly* newsletter. (September) 10(2).

"Untie the elderly." The Kendal Corporation, PO Box 100, Kennett Square, PA 19348. www.ute.kendal.org

Williams CC, Burger SG, Murphy K. 1997. Restraint reduction. In Morris JN, Lipsitz LA, Murphy KM, Belleville-Taylor P, eds. *Quality care in the nursing home.* St. Louis, MO: Mosby.

Authors

Beryl D. Goldman, PhD, RN
Neil Beresin, MEd, BA
Janet Davis, BA, ACC
Harriet Finne-Soveri, MD, PhD
Brant E. Fries, PhD
John P. Hirdes, PhD
Karen Russell, LPN
Sara Wright, MSN, GNP
Katharine M. Murphy, PhD, RN
John N. Morris, PhD, MSW
Knight Steel, MD

Part II

Cognition/Mental Health CAPs

Cognitive Loss CAP

Problem

The cognitive hallmarks of an independent life include the ability to remember recent events and the ability to make safe daily decisions. The aging process may be associated with mild impairment. Otherwise, the decline in cognition is likely the result of other factors such as delirium, a mental health problem, a mass lesion, a stroke, a metabolic condition, or dementia.

Dementia is not a unique disease, but a syndrome. It may be linked to several causes. According to DSM-IV-TR, the dementia syndrome is defined by the presence of three criteria:*

- a short-term memory problem,

- **and** trouble with at least one cognitive function (abstract thought, judgment, orientation, language, behavior, personality change, and so on),

- **and** these troubles have an impact on the performance of daily life activities.

Declining or worsening cognitive abilities threaten personal independence and increase the risk for long-term care facility admission. Whatever the reason for cognitive decline, care based on a proper diagnosis is necessary for proper planning.

Overall Goals of Care

- Optimize the ability to perform activities of daily living and to live an active social life.

- Prevent further cognitive and physical decline.

- Support safe and independent decision making.

Cognitive Loss CAP Trigger

This CAP focuses on helping persons with reasonable cognitive skills, characterized by a CPS score of 2 or lower (corresponding to a Mini-Mental State Examination [MMSE] score of 19 or higher), to remain as independent as possible, for as long as possible. It triggers for focused care planning the subgroup of persons who are at higher risk of losing their retained cognitive abilities. These persons will have, or will be at risk of having, a form of dementia. Loss of instrumental or basic activities of daily living (ADL) function, in the absence of a physical illness, should raise

---

*The notion of decline and chronicity should also be considered: (1) if there is a decline but without the presence of the three criteria together that are described above, one can talk of cognitive impairment or cognitive loss; (2) if the troubles are not chronic but fluctuating, a delirium is more probably involved.

suspicion of emerging cognitive impairment. Therefore, careful observation of a person's performance of these activities over time may provide an important clue to suggest the presence of cognitive decline.

TRIGGERED TO PREVENT DECLINE

This group includes persons who exhibit **both** of the following:

- Cognitive Performance Scale (CPS) score of 0, 1, or 2 (equivalent to a MMSE of 19 or higher), **and**

- The presence of two or more of the following clinical risk factors for cognitive decline:

  - Alzheimer's disease

  - Dementia other than Alzheimer's disease

  - Sometimes or never/rarely able to understand others

  - Sometimes or never/rarely able to make self understood

  - Repetitive daily complaints or concerns

  - Repetitive questions

  - Repetitive daily verbalization that something bad is about to happen

  - Wandering

  - Physically abusive

  - New indications of being easily distracted—this element is not assessed in RAI-HC

  - New episodes of altered perception — this element is not assessed in RAI-HC

  - New episodes of disorganized speech — this element is not assessed in RAI-HC

  - New periods of restlessness — this element is not assessed in RAI-HC

  - New periods of lethargy — this element is not assessed in RAI-HC

  - New indication that mental function varies over the course of the day (sudden change in mental function)

  - Declining cognitive status over the past 90 days (or worsening decision making as compared to status of 90 days ago is different than declining cognitive status over the past 90 days)*

  - Increased care needs over the past 90 days (in P6–CS ask participants to remove "receives more support" in code 2 and tell them to focus on the word "deterioration")

  - Six or fewer months to live

These persons have early indications of cognitive problems and are at a higher risk of declining further in the near future. This group includes about 5% of persons in long-term care facilities, 10% of persons receiving home care, and less than 1% of older adults living independently in the community. In a long-term care facility setting, about 25% of the persons triggered into this group will experience a decline in cognition over a 90-day period (with proportional declines in memory and independence in daily decision making). The rate of decline in home care is about 16%.

---

*This parenthetical criteria applies when the loneliness item is not available on the instrument.

TRIGGERED TO MONITOR FOR RISK OF COGNITIVE DECLINE

This group includes persons who exhibit **both** of the following:

- Cognitive Performance Scale (CPS) score of 0, 1, or 2 (equivalent to a MMSE score of 19 or higher), and

- The presence of **none or only one** of the previously mentioned risk factors for cognitive decline (listed under "Triggered to prevent decline").

These persons tend to decline as they subsequently acquire two or more of the risk factors. **The approach to care for these persons is to observe their performance for the onset of these factors.**

This group includes about 35% of persons in long-term care facilities, 75% of persons receiving home care, and 98% of older adults living independently in the community. In a long-term care home setting, about 13% of the persons triggered into this group will tend to decline in cognitive performance over a 90-day period. The rate of decline in home care tends to be about 10%.

NOT TRIGGERED

Includes all persons with a Cognitive Performance Scale (CPS) score of 3 or higher (equivalent to a MMSE score lower than 19).

This group includes about 60% of persons in long-term care facilities, 15% of persons receiving home care, and 1% of older adults living independently in the community. In both long-term care facility and home care settings, only about 8% of persons in this group tend to experience a decline in cognitive performance over a 90-day period.

Cognitive Loss CAP Guidelines

Initial Diagnostic Workup When There Is No Dementia Diagnosis Present

It is possible for a person to be in the early stages of dementia, even though the CPS score is low. If there is suspicion of cognitive impairment, it is recommended that further evaluation be completed and referrals put in place. In cases where the information provided by the person or family members is unclear, it may be necessary to consult the physician directly.

Persons without a known diagnosis of dementia should be considered for referral to a physician for further assessment when

- The CPS score is 1 or 2 **or** 0 but there is other evidence of cognitive impairment (for example, a recent cognitive loss). In such a case, persons who do not have a proper explanation for their decline in cognition function should have a comprehensive medical evaluation to rule out (or in) treatable reasons for cognitive impairment and to identify optimal medications.

- Other evidence of cognitive impairment includes the symptoms listed in the "clinical risk factors" referenced under the triggers. It might also include reduced performance in instrumental and basic ADLs that is not explained by a physical illness or impairment.

If the need for assistance is still unclear, consult a physician. Review the person's clinical records and most recent interRAI assessments for possible reasons, other than impaired cognition, that are contributing to this need for assistance in ADLs. These might include

Physiological disorders, for example:

- Musculoskeletal diseases

- Neurological diseases

■ Post-trauma conditions

Factors associated with lifestyle and adopted habits, for example:

■ Excessive use of alcohol

■ Use of psychotropic medications [see Appropriate Medications CAP]

■ Household roles (for example, in many relationships, partners may assume responsibilities for specific tasks such as housekeeping and managing finances)

If the need for assistance is still unclear, consult a physician. Even if a reasonable explanation for impaired performance is found, continue to observe for signs of declining cognition or physical performance.

However, all persons with a CPS of 1 or 2 who do not have a proper explanation should have a comprehensive medical evaluation to rule out (or in) treatable reasons for cognitive impairment and to identify optimal medications.

The assessment follow-up may range from a single consultation with a physician to a comprehensive process involving neuropsychological testing, haematologic investigations, and brain imaging.

Look for Reversible Causes of Cognitive Loss

Almost any new medication can have a negative impact on cognition. [See Appropriate Medications CAP.]

Some types of cognitive loss, such as those due to low levels of serum vitamin B12, disorders in calcium metabolism or thyroid function, or excessive use of alcoholic beverages, may be reversible. For those triggered to prevent cognitive decline, review the following clinical risk factors for possible links to subsequent cognitive loss.

Signs of fluctuating cognitive status. Delirium, or acute confusion, is a potentially reversible condition. However, it can result in the wrong impression about the nature of the person's typical or usual cognitive limitation. Improved cognitive performance can be expected in many persons as delirium resolves. [See Delirium CAP.]

For persons with a diagnosis of any dementing disease, assess for signs of declining cognitive performance.

■ Caregivers should be asked to identify potentially reversible causes (other than the dementia-causing disease itself) for recent losses in cognitive status. The actions of caregivers and family may overly compensate for a modest decline in function. The goal is to allow the person to make maximal use of retained cognitive abilities in daily life. It would be incorrect to assume that recent loss of this type is not reversible.

■ Identifying these changes can heighten caregiver awareness of the person's cognitive and functional limitations, while offering an opportunity to re-engage the person in making decisions and performing everyday activities of daily life. Knowledge of cognitive decline will help others develop practical expectations of the person's capabilities and aid in designing approaches to maximize the person's involvement in making daily decisions.

Are there behavioral symptoms (for example, wandering or physical abuse of others) that interfere with daily life, care delivery, or activities involvement? [See Behavior CAP.]

■ Specific treatments for behavioral problems and treatments for delirium may effectively address these conditions and improve cognitive capabilities. [See Delirium CAP and Behavior CAP.]

- Pain has a negative impact on cognition. Pain in persons with impaired cognition can also cause behavioral problems, irritability, and function loss. [See Pain CAP.]

- Some behavior problems will not be reversible. [See Behavior CAP.] If this is the case, and the behaviors occur daily, another environment for the person might be appropriate. However, in the mild stages of cognitive impairment, the person should be able to make many of his or her own life decisions, including where to live.

- Some behavior problems may pose no threat to the person's safety, health, or activity pattern or the safety of others and do not require intervention. But if there is a temporal relationship between behavior and cognitive decline, consider treating the behavior. The following issues may be considered:
  - Have cognitive skills declined after beginning a behavior management program (for example, psychotropic drugs)?
  - Is the decline due to the treatment program (for example, a side effect of a drug)?
  - Have cognitive skills improved following the onset of a behavioral management program?
  - Has caregiver help strengthened the person's self-performance patterns?

Does the person suffer from symptoms of depression?

- Depressive symptoms may cause a cognitive decline that is mistakenly interpreted as dementia. [See Mood CAP.]

Are there other medical problems?

- Identifying and treating other medical problems may improve cognitive functioning and a person's quality of life. For example, therapy for congestive heart failure or chronic obstructive pulmonary disease may lead to functional and cognitive improvement, while conditions such as chronic liver disease and renal failure can cause or worsen a cognitive loss. These conditions are almost always under a physician's care. Thus, if the person begins to experience a new cognitive loss, discuss with the physician the possibility of a relationship to these conditions or a new or changed treatment for them.

- An increase in pain can lead to decreased involvement in functional activities, and this mistakenly may be assumed to indicate cognitive decline. [See Pain CAP.]

Can the person communicate effectively with others? Many persons suffering from cognitive deficits seem incapable of full meaningful communication. As a result, seemingly incomprehensible behaviors (for example, screaming) may represent a person's only form of communication. [See Communication CAP.] Be certain that the failure to communicate effectively is not due to hearing impairment or a neurological deficit (for example, aphasia).

- Speak with the caregiver and family about the best methods of communicating with the person. Sometimes it will be these individuals who best understand how to make contact with the person; in other instances, they will need help in adopting a new approach for the person who has recently declined.

- Is the person willing or able to engage in meaningful communication?

- Does the caregiver use nonverbal communication techniques (for example, touch, gesture) to encourage the person to respond?

Review the person's medication record for drug(s) that might affect cognition. Consider a discussion with the physician or a referral to a consulting pharmacist to aid in this review.

- Many medications, particularly psychoactive drugs, may cause cognitive decline. [See Appropriate Medications CAP.]

- A person may show a sudden decline in cognitive function because a drug has been either started or stopped. A thorough review of the medication record, including both prescribed and over-the-counter drugs, will help to identify any recent change in drug consumption practice.

- Some medications may be marginally helpful in preventing a decline in cognitive status in some people with Alzheimer's disease. If these medications are not being taken, or have never been tried, discuss this option with the physician.

- Be alert for evidence of chronic or acute alcohol ingestion or the use of street drugs.

- Be alert for the use of herbal remedies or alternative medications the person might be taking.

Continued Involvement in Daily Life

Are there opportunities for independent activity? Decline in one functional area neither signals the need for the caregiver to assume full responsibility in that area nor should it be interpreted as an indication of a definitive decline in other areas. Review information in the assessment while considering the following issues:

- Are there factors that suggest the person can be more involved in his or her care (for example, instances of greater self-performance; wish to do more independently; retained ability to learn; retained control over trunk, limbs, or hands)?

- Can the person participate more in decisions about daily life?

- Does the person retain any cognitive ability that would allow greater involvement in decision making?

- Is the person passive?

- Does the person resist care?

- Are activities broken into manageable subtasks?

What is the extent and rate of change of the person's functional abilities? Functional changes are often the first indicators of cognitive decline and suggest the need to identify reversible causes. [See IADL CAP and ADL CAP.] Consider the following:

- To what extent is the person dependent in locomotion, dressing, and eating?

- Are there problems with standing balance and risk for falls? [See Falls CAP.]

- Could the person be more independent with appropriate cueing or restorative programming?

- Nutritional status and weight loss are associated with decline in physical function and may prevent physical improvement. [See ADL CAP and Undernutrition CAP.]

- Would an appropriate referral prevent further decline?

What is the person's extent of continued involvement in ADLs and daily life? Programs focused on physical and social aspects of the person's life can sometimes lessen the disruptive symptoms of cognitive decline. Consider the following:

- Can adjusting task demands or the environmental circumstances under which tasks are carried out be helpful?

- Are small group programs encouraged?

- Are special environmental stimuli present (for example, directional markers, special lighting, color coding)?

- Do caregivers regularly help the person in ways that permit him or her to maintain or attain the highest level of functioning? For example, are verbal reminders, physical cues, and supervision regularly provided to aid in carrying out ADLs; are ADL tasks presented in segments to give the person enough time to respond to cues; and is assistance provided in a pleasant and encouraging manner?

- Has the person experienced a recent loss of someone close (for example, the death of a spouse, a change in the primary caregiver, a recent move to a more dependent living environment, or decreased visiting by family and friends)?

Is the person experiencing a failure to thrive? There is a point at which the accumulated health and neurological problems of cognitively impaired persons can place them at an elevated risk of complications (for example, pressure ulcers) as well as death. As this disability approaches, review the following:

- Do emotional, social, or environmental factors play key roles in the management of these problems?

- If a person is not eating, to what can it be attributed? Examples include a reversible mood problem, a negative reaction to the physical and social environment in which eating activity occurs, or a neurological deficit such as the loss of hand coordination that might be overcome with specially designed utensils.

- Can an identified problem be corrected through caregiver education, a trial of antidepressant medication, referral to occupational therapy (OT) for training, or a counseling program?

- If a cause cannot be identified, what clinical conditions may be reversible or preventable as death approaches (for example, fecal impaction, pain, and pressure ulcers)? What interventions could prevent, or at least decrease, the likelihood of such complications?

Persons with developmental disabilities. Increasing numbers of persons with developmental disabilities live longer lives. Some may develop dementia as they age. With declining cognition, families and other caregivers may have to adjust the living environment or other aspects of the person's life to help him or her live as independently as possible.

Note that many of the above guidelines also are helpful when care planning for those with a CPS score of 3 or higher.

Additional Resources

Mace N, Morris JN, Lombardo NE, Perls T. 1997. Cognitive loss. In Morris JN, Lipsitz LA, Murphy KM, Belleville-Taylor P, eds. *Quality care in the nursing home.* St. Louis, MO: Mosby.

The Web site maintained by the Alzheimer's Association (www.alz.org) is an excellent resource. It contains much information, including lists of recent articles, books, and videos, a summary of tips for caregivers, and links to many other Web sites (such as www.alzheimer.ca).

Authors

John N. Morris, PhD, MSW
Harriet Finne-Soveri, MD, PhD
Katharine M. Murphy, PhD, RN
Knight Steel, MD
Pauline Belleville-Taylor, RN, MS, CS

Delirium CAP

Problem

The Delirium CAP focuses on issues of delirium (acute cognitive loss) and the related differential diagnosis of chronic cognitive loss and dementia. Identifying problems and their intertwined causation is central to person's lives. The notions of decline and chronicity need to be taken into account. If the troubles are fluctuating or of recent onset, it is more probable that the issue to be addressed is delirium.

Delirium is a serious condition that is usually caused by an underlying acute health problem such as an infection, dehydration, or drug reaction. It is associated with high mortality and morbidity (for example, development of pressure ulcers, functional decline, persistence of behavioral symptoms, hospitalization). This CAP presents an approach to addressing the needs of persons who present with these symptoms.

Delirium is common among inpatients or those recently discharged from a health care setting, including large numbers with pre-existing cognitive impairment. Approximately 25% of persons admitted to a long-term care facility from an acute-care setting will have a measure of delirium that restricts their success in rehabilitation and prolongs their stay. Rates increase from 25% to 80–90% among persons who are at the end of life, causing discomfort for the dying person and his or her family.

Early recognition and treatment of delirium is crucial. Clinicians who are in regular contact with the person are in the best position to recognize, assess, and collaborate with physicians and other primary care providers in instituting a plan of care.

Delirium is never part of normal aging. Some of its classic signs are often mistaken for the progression of dementia, particularly in the later stages of this condition. Unlike dementia, delirium has a rapid onset (hours to days). Typical signs include difficulty paying attention; fluctuating behavior or cognitive function throughout the day; restlessness; sleepiness during the day; rambling; nonsensical speech; and altered perceptions, such as misinterpretations (illusion), seeing or feeling things that are not there (hallucination), or a fixed false belief (delusion).

Successful management depends on an accurate identification of the clinical condition, correct diagnosis of specific cause(s), and prompt nursing and medical intervention. Delirium is often caused and aggravated by multiple factors. If one cause is identified and addressed, but delirium continues, reassess for other potential causes. The focus is on addressing the underlying clinical problems such as treating infections, addressing dehydration, relieving pain and depression, managing medications, ensuring optimal sensory input (for example, with the use of glasses and hearing aids), and promoting as normal as possible the social and functional status in the environment within which the person is staying.

Even when the delirium is identified and interventions are implemented in the hospital setting, the delirium often will still be present when the person is discharged to another setting (for example, home, a long-term care facility, or supportive housing). Both family and formal caregivers need to be aware of interventions that have been successful in starting to reverse the delirium. Family members and caregivers must ensure the person's safety in the home. A person discharged home while still in a delirious state should not be driving a car or operating machinery and should not be responsible for the care of others while in the delirious state.

In some cases, the person will not be able to be left alone due to safety issues, and will need supervision in taking medications, cooking, and other ADLs. Discharging staff should discuss this with the person and his or her family. Staff can be instrumental in helping family support any activity restrictions until the person's delirium has cleared.

Overall Goals of Care

- Identify and treat underlying cause(s) of delirium.

- Monitor and care for delirium symptoms and other delirium-related health, mood, and behavioral symptoms (for example, pulling out tubes, unsafe climbing).

- Prevent secondary complications (for example, those associated with physical restraints, falls, dehydration, inappropriate use of psychotropic drugs that may cause or exacerbate delirium).

- Prevent a recurrence of delirium.

Delirium CAP Trigger

This CAP is triggered when a person has active symptoms of delirium. The goal of treatment is to return the person to his or her baseline status.

TRIGGERED

This group includes persons who exhibit any of the following symptoms:

interRAI Suite Assessment tools (LTCF, HC)

- Behavior in the following areas appears different from usual functioning, either new onset or worsening or different from recent times: easily distracted, episodes of disorganized speech, mental function varies over the course of the day.

- Acute change in mental status from person's usual functioning.

MDS 2.0

- Behavior present over the last 7 days appears different than the person's usual functioning: easily distracted, periods of altered perception or awareness of surroundings, episodes of disorganized speech, periods of restlessness, periods of lethargy, mental function that varies over the course of the day.

- Sudden or new onset change in mental function over the last 7 days.

This triggered group includes about 1 to 20% of persons in long-term care facilities, 3 to 15% of persons receiving home care, and less than 1% of older persons living independently in the community.

NOT TRIGGERED

This group includes persons who have none of the previously noted symptoms.

Physician Communication and Involvement in Assessment and Care Planning

Initial management. Assessment and initial treatment of delirium rests with nursing staff and physicians. When this CAP is triggered, it suggests that the person may have delirium. Referral to an appropriately qualified health professional, proficient in the diagnosis of delirium, is an important first step in responding to this triggered CAP.

However, if it is not possible to secure a referral within hours, it should be assumed that delirium is present and the person's care should be managed accordingly, while waiting for further advice.

To coordinate effective care approaches, nurses must be prepared to communicate signs of delirium, CAP guideline assessment findings, and concerns to the physician. The more thorough and factual the communication with the physician, the easier it will be to determine an appropriate course of action in a timely fashion. The absence of significant findings should also be communicated to the physician. For example, observations that the person has stable vital signs, has no fever, has no obvious signs of infection or dehydration, has been eating and drinking adequately, and has been receiving no new drugs will help to formulate the next course of action.

Nursing Observations

Changes in vital signs:

- Take and record vital signs (temperature, pulse, respiration, and blood pressure).

- Compare these vital signs to the person's usual/baseline pattern. The following measures are clinically significant and should prompt an evaluation for possible causes:

  - Rectal temperatures above 100° F (38° C) or below 95° F (35° C).

  - Pulse rate less than 60 or greater than 100 beats per minute.

  - Respiratory rate over 25 breaths per minute, or less than 16 per minute. For accuracy, count breaths for 1 full minute.

  - Hypotension or a significant decrease in blood pressure:
    - a systolic blood pressure of less than 90 mm Hg, **or**
    - a decline of 20 mm Hg or greater in systolic blood pressure from the person's usual baseline, **or**
    - a decline of 10 mm Hg or greater in diastolic blood pressure from the person's usual baseline.

  - Hypertension:
    - a systolic blood pressure above 160 mm Hg, **or**
    - a diastolic blood pressure above 95 mm Hg.

Signs of infection:

- Fever suggesting a possible urinary tract infection, pneumonia, or other infection.

- Because fever may be absent in an immunocompromised person with an infection, pay attention to other signs, including cloudy or foul-smelling urine, congested lungs or cough, dyspnea, diarrhea, abdominal pain, purulent wound drainage, or erythema (redness) around an incision.

Indicators of dehydration. [See Dehydration CAP.] If the Dehydration CAP is triggered, proceed under the assumption that this is a problem. If it is not triggered, the following review may help to identify persons not identified by that CAP.

- Recent decrease in urine volume or more concentrated urine than usual

- Recent decrease in eating habits — skipping meals or leaving food uneaten, weight loss

- Nausea, vomiting, diarrhea, or blood loss

- Receiving intravenous drugs

- Receiving diuretics or drugs that may cause electrolyte imbalance

Person in pain. [See Pain CAP.]

- Review pain frequency, intensity, and characteristics (time of onset, duration, quality).

- If the person is receiving an analgesic (pain medication), is the dosing adequate to avoid pain breakthrough? If the analgesic is suspected as the cause of the delirium, the person should have a trial on another analgesic medication from a different drug classification.

Are there indicators of a flare-up of a known chronic condition? Common problems include the following:

- Congestive heart failure

- Diabetes

    - Signs of hypoglycemia include weakness, sweating, tachycardia, nervousness, hunger, and headache.

    - Signs of hyperglycemia include weakness, thirst, greater urine output than usual, and confusion.

- Emphysema/COPD with shortness of breath, wheezing

- CVA (stroke) or TIA (transient ischemic attack): any **new** slurring of speech, limb weakness or numbness, vision changes, new or worsening incontinence, new facial asymmetry

- Thyroid disease

- Gastrointestinal bleeding

- Review any recent changes in physician orders and new laboratory values

Signs of recent functional decline. [See ADL CAP.]

- Recent decline in overall ADL status — assess why ADLs have declined and the likelihood of recovery following reversal of the delirium.

    - Is the ADL decline secondary to delirium?

- In what ADL area(s) is the decline present — hygiene, locomotion, eating?

    - Are there associated falls? [See Falls CAP.]

Drug Review

Review the medications the person is taking to identify drugs or regimens that might be associated with delirium. A consulting pharmacist can be invaluable in this review.

- Is (are) there new medication(s) or dosage increase(s)? Review the length of time from medication change(s) to the onset of symptoms. The person could have been on delirium- inducing medications while in acute care and the effects may still be present on discharge to a subacute unit or long- term care facility.

- Is there any specific medication known to contribute to delirium? Almost any drug can cause delirium, but common medications include

  - Drugs with anticholinergic properties (for example, some antipsychotics, antidepressants, antiparkinsonian drugs, antihistamines)

  - Opioids (narcotic pain drug), especially Demerol (meperidine), which is often used postsurgically

  - Benzodiazepines, especially long-acting agents

  - Recent abrupt discontinuation, omission, or decrease in dose of short- or long-acting benzodiazepines. Benzodiazepine withdrawal is important to consider in recent (re)admissions from home, hospital, or other institution.

  - Drug interactions (pharmacist review may be required)

  - It is important to note that drug errors or adverse drug reactions resulting from drug or dosage changes (intended or inadvertent) during transfer from hospital to a long-term care facility are a common problem in older persons. Communication with the hospital to minimize these problems may be critical.

- Is the person taking more than one drug from a particular class of drugs? A pharmacist may be helpful in this review.

- Consider drug toxicity, especially if the person is dehydrated or has renal insufficiency. Does the person have a history of drug toxicity? Review the record. Serum drug level should be considered for some drugs.

Monitor for Associated or Progressive Signs and Symptoms

- Sleep disturbances (for example, up and awake at night/asleep during the day)

- Agitation and inappropriate movements (for example, unsafe climbing out of bed or chair, pulling out tubes). In these situations, the person may need one-on-one supervision. Physical restraint should only be considered as a last resort and only if it is clinically justified (for example, if the person needs a lifesaving drug or fluid via intravenous tube and restraint alternatives, such as diversion, are ineffective). [See Restraint CAP.]

- Motor hypoactivity (for example, low or lack of motor activity, lethargy, or sluggish responses), increasing the risk of aspiration and pressure ulcers

- Perceptual disturbances common to drug withdrawal such as hallucinations (seeing or feeling things not present) and delusions (for example, mistaking a blowing curtain for a person climbing in a window)

Other Considerations

Psychosocial issues to consider:

- Any recent change in mood (for example, crying, social withdrawal). Remember that delirium is often a frightening experience for the person. He or she needs reminders that the condition is temporary.

- Any recent change in social situation (for example, isolation, recent loss of family member or friend). For persons who have experienced an environmental change, first rule out other causes of delirium.

Physical or environmental factors that could make confusion worse:

- Is the person's hearing or vision impaired? Impairment may have an impact on the person's ability to process information (directions, reminders, environmental cues). Make sure the person uses his or her glasses or hearing aids (if usually worn).

- Is the person **not** receiving frequent reorientation, reassurance, or reminders to help him or her make sense of things?

- Has there been a recent change in environment (for example, an intensive care unit stay, room or unit change, new admission, or return from hospital)? Avoid moving the person to a new setting unless indicated clinically.

- Is there anything that is interfering with the person's ability to get enough sleep (for example, light, noise, frequent disruptions)?

- Is the environment noisy or chaotic (for example, calling out, loud music, constant commotion, frequent caregiver changes)?

End of life considerations. Delirium is common at the end of life. However, it is not usually appropriate to begin an aggressive or invasive work-up to identify the cause(s) of delirium in persons who are actively dying or who have orders for "comfort measures only." A more focused evaluation to determine if current palliative measures are adequate in managing the person's, family's, or unit's (for example, the person is very noisy) comfort is warranted. Discussion with the family is key to establishing goals for care. A balance must be sought between the degree of pain control and the level of consciousness desired. The goals and approach of care should be directed to achieving maximum comfort. Consider the following:

- **Is the person in pain?** An increased dose or frequency of administration or a stronger or additional analgesic may be warranted.

- **Are the person's medications contributing to the delirium?** The drug review should emphasize opioids (narcotics), neuroleptics (antipsychotics), antiepileptics, nonsteroidal anti-inflammatory agents and other pain relievers, antibiotics, and drugs for constipation and diarrhea.

  - Would the person be more comfortable without the drug or with a lower dose, or does the benefit of comfort from the drug outweigh the side effect of delirium?

- **Does the person have "terminal agitation" (uncontrollable delirium)?** Sedation may be warranted to decrease fear and suffering and prevent accidental injury.

Additional Resources

American Psychiatric Association (APA). 2004. Practice guideline for treatment of patients with delirium. *American Journal of Psychiatry* (May). **Note:** This guideline provides a detailed general overview of the delirium syndrome and the role of the psychiatrist in delirium management. These guidelines are also available at the APA Web site: www.psych.org (click on "Clinical Resources" and then click on "Practice Guidelines"). This site also includes Patient and Family Guides that would also be useful in training nurse assistants.

American Psychiatric Association (APA). 2004. Practice guideline for treatment of patients with delirium. *American Journal of Psychiatry* (August).

Flacker JM, Marcantonio ER. 1998. Delirium in the elderly: Optimal management. *Drugs and Aging* 13: 119–30. **Note:** This article provides a detailed approach to treatment and monitoring of delirium.

Inouye SK. 2006. Current concepts: Delirium in older persons. *N Engl J Med.* 354: 1157–65.

Murphy KM, Levkoff S, Lipsitz LA. 1997. Delirium. In Morris JN, Lipsitz LA, Murphy KM, Belleville-Taylor P, eds. *Quality care in the nursing home.* St. Louis, MO: Mosby. **Note:** This chapter provides an overview of the syndrome particularly as it affects nursing home persons and staff. Detailed nonpharmacologic approaches and case examples are presented.

Rapp CG. 1999. Acute confusion/delirium (evidence-based protocol). The Iowa Veterans Affairs Nursing Research Consortium, University of Iowa Gerontological Nursing Interventions Center. **Note:** This protocol provides helpful information for developing a comprehensive care plan for persons with delirium. www.nursing.uiowa.edu

---

Authors

Katharine M. Murphy, PhD, RN
Edward Marcantonio, MD
Sharon K. Inouye, MD
John N. Morris, PhD, MSW

Communication CAP

Problem

While many conditions can affect how a person expresses and comprehends information, the Communication CAP focuses on the interplay between the person's communication status and his or her cognitive skills for everyday decision making. Normal communication involves two related activities:

- Expressive communication: Making oneself understood to others, usually verbally but also through nonverbal exchange. Typical expressive problems include disruptions in language, speech, and voice production. Specific manifestations include difficulty in finding suitable words, putting a sentence together, or describing objects and events; pronouncing words incorrectly; stuttering; hoarse or distorted voice; and low volume because of poor respiratory status. The percentage of persons with at least some difficulty in making themselves understood ranges from 15% of those living independently in the community, to 25% of those receiving home care, to 40% of persons in long-term care facilities.

- Receptive communication: Comprehending or understanding the verbal or written communication of others. Typical receptive communication problems include changes/difficulties in hearing, speech discrimination, vocabulary comprehension, reading, and interpreting facial expressions. The percentage of persons with at least some difficulty in comprehending the verbal communication of others ranges from 10% for those living in the community, to 25% of persons receiving home care, to 50% of persons in long-term care facilities.

Overall Goals of Care

- Prevent avoidable loss of communication skills for as long as possible.

- Reverse or improve communication loss.

- Monitor a list of common causal factors and treat as appropriate.

- Work with families and caregivers to ensure effective communication with the person.

Communication CAP Trigger

The goal of this CAP is twofold: first, to work to improve communication ability whenever possible; and second, to prevent avoidable communication decline. Anyone triggered should receive a specialized communication care plan follow-up. The key difference between the following two triggered groups is whether the goal of care is improvement or preventing decline.

TRIGGERED TO FACILITATE IMPROVEMENT

This subgroup is defined by the presence of both of two factors:

- Moderate to severe communication shortfalls, which include both communication with others and understanding communication from others; and

- Some ability to engage in everyday decision making (a measure of cognitive reserve).

Given these cognitive abilities, persons in this subgroup are the most likely to experience improvements in communication. Yet, only a minority (about 15%) will improve over the ensuing 90-day period, and the principal focus of care is to increase the likelihood of this happening. Note that this group includes about 11% of persons in long-term care facilities, 8% of persons receiving home care, and less than 1% of older adults living independently in the community.

TRIGGERED TO PREVENT DECLINE

This subgroup is also defined by a person's communication and everyday decision-making ability, but in this instance the person has better baseline communication skills and poorer everyday decision-making capability.

Given the absence of cognitive reserves, this subgroup is the most likely to decline in communication. Yet, only a minority will decline (about 15%), and the principal focus of care is to reduce the likelihood of this happening. Note that this group includes about 25% of persons in long-term care facilities, 10% of persons receiving home care, and less than 1% of older adults living independently in the community.

NOT TRIGGERED

This subgroup includes anyone for whom either functional recovery or functional maintenance to prevent decline is not a clinically realistic care goal. There is a balance between communication skills and cognitive ability (as measured by everyday decision making). There are three such groupings: good communication and good cognition, middle communication and middle cognition, and poor communication and poor cognition.

This subgroup is the least likely to change over time, as communication ability matches cognitive ability. Note that this group includes about 64% of persons in long-term care facilities, 88% of persons receiving home care, and 99% of older adults living independently in the community. Care for persons in this group is limited to monitoring for any unexpected decline in communication levels.

Communication CAP Guidelines

When communication is limited, assessment focuses on reviewing several factors: underlying causes of the deficit, the success of attempted remedial actions, the person's ability to compensate with nonverbal strategies (for example, ability to visually follow nonverbal signs and signals), and the willingness and ability of caregivers to ensure effective communication. In the presence of reduced language skills, both caregivers and the person must expand their nonverbal communication skills — one of the most basic and automatic of human abilities. Touch, facial expression, eye contact, hand movements, tone of voice, and posture are all powerful means of communicating. Recognizing and using all practical means is the key to effective communication.

Assess the person for confounding problems and address them. [See relevant CAPs.] As these confounding problems lessen or further decline is prevented, the person's communication abilities should be reviewed.

- Decline in cognitive status, especially recent onset of acute confusion (delirium)

- Increased number of mood indicators (for example, an increase on the Depression Rating Scale [DRS])

- Decline in ADL status

- Deterioration in respiratory status in persons with COPD

- Oral motor function — swallowing, clarity of voice production

Assess and correct, where possible, the components of communication. Details of the person's strengths and weaknesses in understanding, hearing, and expression are part of a supportive treatment program.

- Hearing impairment: Check that proper hearing appliance is present, operating correctly (for example, batteries are working), and is being used. Determine if the person is able to understand in particular situations, for example, in a quiet environment or when talking one-on-one where he or she can see the other's lips.

- Communication success: If the person is able to communicate more effectively with certain individuals, then try to determine why this is the case. For example, does the person speak slowly and distinctly, use specific gestures or motions, or communicate in another language? Ensure provision of this effective mode of communication.

- Nonverbal communication: If the person has the capacity to use communication devices or other nonverbal modes of communication, ensure that the staff and/or caregiver is aware of the need to employ such procedures and is trained in their use.

- Recent decline in hearing: Review for potential causes, including presence of ear discharge(s) and cerumen (wax) accumulation.

Review treatment and evaluation history:

- Has the person received an evaluation by an audiologist or Speech-Language Pathologist (SLP)? How recently?

- Has the person's condition worsened since the most recent evaluation?

- If such an evaluation resulted in a plan of care, has it been followed as specified?

Factors to be assessed and addressed for possible relationship to communication problems:

- **Recent onset conditions** (for example, aphasia secondary to stroke). If improvement is possible, consider referral to a SLP.

- **Chronic or recurrent conditions** (for example, Alzheimer's disease or other dementia, aphasia following a stroke, Parkinson's disease, mental health problem). For chronic conditions that are unlikely to improve with treatment, consider communication interventions that might compensate for losses (for example, for moderately impaired persons with Alzheimer's disease, the use of short, direct phrases and tactile approaches to communication can be effective).

- **Conditions that may display voice production deficits** (for example, asthma, emphysema/COPD, Parkinson's disease, cancer, or poorly fitting dentures). Consider a consultation with a physical therapist for breathing exercises or cardiorespiratory endurance training, physician, or dentist.

- **Transitory conditions** (for example, delirium, infection(s), or an acute illness). Are there acute or transitory conditions, which if successfully resolved might result in an improved ability to communicate? [See Delirium CAP or refer to physician.]

- **Assess the person's drug regimen for conditions that could impair his or her ability to communicate.** Would drug titration or substitution result in an improved ability to communicate? Consult with the physician when the following medications are used:

  - Psychotropic medications such as antidepressant agents and tranquilizing agents (including antipsychotic, anti-anxiety, and sedative agents)

  - Opioid (narcotic) analgesics

  - Antiparkinsonian medications

  - Antibiotics such as gentamycin and tobramycin

  - Aspirin

- **Assess the person's opportunities to communicate where the quality and quantity of communication are equal to apparent ability.** Are opportunities to communicate limited in ways that could be corrected (for example, the availability of others to communicate with or the use of a communication board or computer)?

Additional Resource

Lubinski R, Frattali C, Barth C. 1997. Communication. In Morris JN, Lipsitz LA, Murphy KM, and Belleville-Taylor P, eds. *Quality care in the nursing home.* St. Louis, MO: Mosby. **Note:** This chapter provides an approach assessment of the person with communication deficits, including how to assess and address underlying problems and tips for care planning.

Authors

Rosemary Lubinski, EdD
Carol Frattali, PhD
John N. Morris, PhD, MSW

Mood CAP

Problem

Mood disorders (for example, depression, sadness, and anxiety) are common problems for adults in the community and in institutional settings. Depression is often underdiagnosed and undertreated. Where symptom rates are low, underdiagnosing must be considered. Left untreated, mood disorders are disabling and associated with high mortality, functional decline, and unnecessary suffering by the person, family, and caregivers. This CAP focuses on identifying depression, with a pre-existing diagnosis or a depressed mood state that requires attention and possible diagnosis.

Overall Goals of Care

- Identify and address any immediate threats to the person's, or other's, safety that is posed by the mood state.
- Identify and treat any underlying conditions that may have caused or contributed to the mood state.
- Implement a treatment for the mood problem.
- Monitor for response to treatment or adverse effects of treatment.

Mood CAP Trigger

There are three levels to the Mood CAP trigger. The triggers are based on the person's Depression Rating Scale (DRS). Note that while other items in the interRAI assessment may assist with further evaluation, the DRS is the best indicator of a potential or actual problem with depression.

TRIGGER RULES FOR THE MOOD CAP

- First, calculate the DRS by adding the person's code response for the following items. In the interRAI suite each item is first recoded such that 0 = 0, 1, 2 = 1, and 3 = 2, creating a scale ranging from 0 to 14.
  - Person made negative statements
  - Persistent anger with self or others
  - Expressions of what appear to be unrealistic fears
  - Repetitive health complaints
  - Repetitive anxious complaints or concerns
  - Sad, pained, or worried facial expressions
  - Crying, tearfulness

In most computer applications, the DRS will already have been programmed into the system.

■ Second, assign the person to a trigger level as follows:

TRIGGERED — HIGH RISK: DRS SCORE OF 3 OR HIGHER

This group includes about 20% of persons in long-term care facilities, 25% of home care recipients, and 5% of older adults living independently in the community. In a long-term care facility setting, about 42% of the persons triggered into this group will improve over a 90-day period. The rate of improvement in home care tends to be about the same.

TRIGGERED — MEDIUM RISK: DRS SCORE OF 1 OR 2

This group includes about 30% of persons in long-term care facilities, 25% of home care recipients, and 5% of older adults living independently in the community. In a long-term care facility setting, about 25% of the persons triggered into this group will improve over a 90-day period. The rate of improvement for home care recipients is the same, about 25%.

NOT TRIGGERED — DRS SCORE OF 0

This group includes about 50% of persons in long-term care facilities, 50% of home care recipients, and 90% of older adults living independently in the community.

Mood CAP Guidelines

Overview of the Approach to the Person with a Mood Disorder

■ **Initial assessment and stabilization.** There is a spectrum of severity of mood disorders, ranging from mild to life threatening. One primary objective of the initial assessment is to determine whether a person has symptoms of a severe mood disorder that place him or her or others at risk for harm. Clinicians must be able to identify when a person is at risk or poses an imminent risk to others and communicate these findings to the appropriate mental health professionals so that interventions to maintain safety can be implemented immediately.

■ **Determination of the nature of the mood disorder.** There are many possible precipitants to the development of mood disorder symptoms, including psychosocial stressors (such as personal loss), relapse of an underlying mental health problem, a medication side effect, or an active medical condition. It is not uncommon for a person to have more than one precipitant. Selection of the appropriate treatment relies heavily on the assessment of factors contributing to the mood problem.

■ **Treatment and monitoring.** There are many possible treatments appropriate to the wide range of mood disorders. The person who receives treatment must be monitored, as treatment (for example, dose of a medication) may need to be adjusted depending on the person's response.

Initial Assessment Observations

Is the person at risk for self-harm?

■ Inquire about suicidal thoughts (that is, "suicidal ideation") and actions:

- Has the person made a suicide plan?

- Has the person attempted suicide in the past?

- Has the person taken any risky actions such as stockpiling pills, saying good-bye to family, giving away possessions, or writing a note?

- Has the person intentionally harmed or tried to harm him- or herself?

- Has the person been refusing to eat or drink? Has the person experienced recent anorexia or weight loss? [See Dehydration CAP and Undernutrition CAP.]

- Has the person been refusing medication or other therapies?

- Observe for impaired judgment or safety awareness (for example, a person with depression can experience a sense of hopelessness and helplessness, which in turn can have a negative impact on judgment and decisions that he or she makes).

Is the person at risk for harming others?

- Observe for increased anger, mood lability, or agitation.

- Inquire if the person feels threatened by others or has thoughts of harming someone else (for example, a person with a mood problem may have delusional thinking, including paranoia).

- Check for weapons (for example, firearms) and objects that could be used as weapons (for example, dinnerware, sharp pencils, or scissors).

Characterize the full spectrum of symptoms of the mood disorder.

- Assess for subjective symptoms of a mood problem by asking the person whether he or she feels depressed. Note that even persons with dementia often can reply adequately when asked.

  - Person reports feeling sad or an absence of pleasurable moments in life.

  - Person reports having no interest in usual activities or complains of feeling too tired to participate. The person may report increased difficulty concentrating on customary activities.

  - Person describes feelings of worthlessness or guilt (for example, a person may complain of feeling like he or she has become a burden to the family).

  - Person reports diminished appetite or a change in sleep habits.

- Observe for the following objective signs of a mood problem:

  - Person displays increased tearfulness or sadness.

  - Sleep disturbance: either difficulty sleeping or increased sleep. Consider keeping a sleep log to accurately track sleep habits.

  - Person's activity level appears low.

  - Person eats poorly and loses weight [see Undernutrition CAP] or eats more than usual.

- Signs and symptoms of mania or hypomania should also be explored for persons who trigger the Mood CAP. This information can assist with the clinical management of the disorder, as it will assist in identifying a depressed mood related to a bipolar disorder. Review for a history of the following indicators:

  - Racing thoughts or euphoria

  - Increased irritability

- Frequent mood changes

  - Pressured speech

  - Flight of ideas

  - Marked decrease in the need for sleep

  - Agitation or hyperactivity

- Attempt to quantify how long the subjective and objective changes have been present.

Inquire whether family or friends of the person have observed a change in mood.

Determination of the Cause of the Mood Disorder

Review the person's medications for drug(s) or regimen(s) that can be associated with mood changes. Large numbers of prescribed or over-the-counter medications can cause mood changes. Request that a pharmacist or physician review the person's full drug regimen. This assessment should focus on (1) whether any drug could be causing or exacerbating the mood disorder; and (2) whether the antidepressant drug prescribed is at a therapeutic dosage for a significant period of time.

- Any new medication(s), or frequency or drug dosage change? Review the length of time from change to onset of symptoms. [See Appropriate Medications CAP.]

- Any specific medication that may be associated with a mood problem? For example, some medications in the following categories have been associated with mood problems:

  - Corticosteroids

  - Cardiac medications

  - Anticholinergics

  - Anticonvulsants

  - Glaucoma medications

  - Antibiotics

  - Chemotherapeutic agents

  - Narcotics

  - Antipsychotics

  - Other drugs, such as interferon and some over-the-counter medications

- Cessation of a medication (for example, corticosteroids or antidepressant medications) may be associated with a mood problem.

New medications are regularly appearing on the market, and some herbal remedies can positively or negatively affect mood.

Is the development of a mood problem associated with a change in the person's medical condition? Check for the presence of

- **Delirium** — This can mimic depression but may be able to be distinguished from depression by the presence of fluctuating levels of consciousness and new or worsening cognitive impairment. [See Delirium CAP.]

- **Infection** — Examine the person for signs of infection including fever, foul-smelling cloudy urine, or purulent sputum.

- **Pain** is often associated with depression, and in these cases assessing and managing both has to be considered. [See Pain CAP.]

- **Other examples of medical conditions** associated with mood problems include thyroid abnormalities, dehydration, metabolic disorders, recent CVA (stroke), dementia, and cancer. [See Cognitive Loss CAP.]

- Consider consulting a physician to diagnose and treat the medical condition.

Is the development of a mood problem associated with any psychosocial changes?

- Any recent change in environment (for example, moving from the life-long home to an apartment in a senior housing complex or into a long-term care facility)?

- Any recent change in relationships (for example, illness or loss of a relative or a friend, or a relative moving out of town)?

- Any recent change in health perception (for example, perception of being seriously ill)?

- Any clinical or functional change that may affect the person's dignity (for example, new or worsening incontinence, communication decline)?

What has been the course of the mood problem?

- Has the change in mood been abrupt or gradual? Mood disorders rarely develop overnight, and a sudden onset may be a clue to an acute medical illness or delirium.

- Has the mood change been constant or has the person's mood fluctuated between extremes?

Does the person have a history of a mood problem?

- Is there a record of a mood disorder or treatment of one in the past?

- Was treatment for a mood disorder changed or discontinued recently?

To what extent do symptoms of anxiety co-occur with the mood disturbance?

- Although distinct disorders, there is the possibility of occurrence of both mood and anxiety disorders.

Treatment and Monitoring

Response to treatment:

- Continue to monitor safety.

  - Monitor for the presence of suicidal feelings. Thoughts of suicide should always be taken seriously. In some persons with depression, the suicide risk may increase during the early treatment phase when the person's energy is restored.

  - Consider referral to a mental health professional.

  - Continue to monitor for signs of dehydration and assess nutritional status.

- Monitor mood state.

  - Is the mood responding to treatment as anticipated?

- Are there signs that the person may be developing a different mood problem? For example, a person with bipolar disorder may cycle into a manic episode when treated for depression.

- Monitor for the onset of treatment side effects.

  - Anticholinergic side effects (for example, delirium, severe constipation, dry mouth, urinary retention, and blurred vision).

  - New sleep disturbance (insomnia, sudden need for less sleep, or daytime drowsiness).

  - Postural hypotension or gait unsteadiness.

  - Confusion (for example, persons treated with electroconvulsive therapy for a mood disorder may experience transient confusion after treatments).

Need for education about the mood disorder and its treatment:

- What are the person's expectations about psychotherapy or counseling?

- What are the person's concerns about the effects and side effects of psychotropic medication? [See Appropriate Medications CAP.]

- What are the person's expectations about the course of recovery? For example, a person may be unaware that several weeks of treatment with an antidepressant medication may be required before symptoms improve.

- Is the person aware that his or her treatment will require ongoing evaluation, titration of drug dosages, and sometimes a change to different medications in order to achieve adequate dosing, optimal treatment effects, and minimal side effects?

- Is the person aware of the need for a maintenance treatment to prevent relapse of the mood problem?

- If the person is receiving home care or lives in an assisted living facility, is he or she aware of community resources to obtain additional information on mood disorders?

Make sure the team, the person, and the family are aware of the planned length of the treatment, the time frame needed for the treatment to be effective, and the potential adverse effects to watch for. [See Appropriate Medications CAP.]

Additional Resources

Alexopoulos GS, Bruce ML, Hull J, Sirey JA, Kakuma T. 1999. Clinical determinants of suicidal ideation and behavior in geriatric depression. *Archives of General Psychiatry* (November). **Note:** This article reports the results of a study to determine risk factors for suicide in the elderly and provides a brief review of the epidemiology of suicide in the elderly.

Block SD. 2000. Assessing and managing depression in the terminally ill person. *Annals of Internal Medicine* (1 February). **Note:** This article, prepared for the End-of-Life Care Consensus Panel of the American College of Physicians — American Society of Internal Medicine, reviews the challenges encountered in the diagnosis and treatment of grief and depression in the terminally ill person. Case examples are used to illustrate points.

Burrows AB, Morris JN, Simon SE, Hirdes JP, Phillips C. 2002. Development of a minimum data set–based depression rating scale for use in nursing homes. *Age and Aging* 29: 165–72.

Satlin A, Murphy KM. 1997. Depression. In Morris JN, Lipsitz LA, Murphy KM, Belleville-Taylor P, eds. *Quality care in the nursing home.* St. Louis, MO: Mosby.

Note: This chapter provides an overview of the risk factors, presenting signs and symptoms, and treatment options for depression in the elderly. Particular attention is given to the relationship between dementia and depression.

Clinical Practice Guidelines

American Psychiatric Association (APA). 1994. Practice guideline for the treatment of patients with bipolar disorder. *American Journal of Psychiatry* (December). **Note:** This guideline uses an approach similar to the depression guideline for the assessment and management of bipolar disorder.

American Psychiatric Association (APA). 2000. Practice guideline for the treatment of patients with major depressive disorder (revision). *American Journal of Psychiatry* (April). **Note:** This guideline provides a detailed general overview of the clinical characteristics of major depression and the treatment options. Flowcharts are used to assist with decision making. These guidelines are also available at the APA Web site: www.psych.org (click on "Clinical Resources" and then click on "Practice Guidelines"). This site includes Patient and Family Guides, which would also be useful in training nursing assistants.

Depression in primary care: Detection and diagnosis. 1993. Vol. 1: Detection and Diagnosis Clinical Practice Guideline #5. AHCPR Publication # 93-0550 (April). (Available online at www.nlm.nih.gov)

Diagnosis and treatment of depression in late life. 1991. NIH Consensus Statement. (November 4-6). 9(3):1–27. (Available on line at www.nlm.nih.gov).

Lebowitz BD, Pearson JL, Schneider LS, et al. 1997. Diagnosis and treatment of depression in late life: Consensus statement update. *JAMA* 278(14): 1186–90. (Available online at www.nlm.nih.gov)

Piven MLS. 1998. Detection of depression in the cognitively intact older adult (research-based protocol). University of Iowa Gerontological Nursing Interventions Research Center, Research Dissemination Core 10. www.nursing.uiowa.edu

Treatment of major depression. 1993. Vol. 2: Treatment of major depression. Clinical Practice Guideline #5. AHCPR Publication #93-0551 (April).

Authors

Eran D. Metzger, MD
Terry Rabinowitz, MD
John N. Morris, PhD, MSW

Behavior CAP

Problem

The Behavior CAP focuses on reversing the daily display of troubling behaviors in the following areas:

- **Wandering** — moving with no rational purpose, seemingly oblivious to needs or safety.

- **Verbal abuse** — threatening, screaming at, or cursing others.

- **Physical abuse** — hitting, shoving, scratching, or sexually abusing others.

- **Socially inappropriate or disruptive behavior** — examples include making disruptive sounds or noises, screaming out, smearing or throwing food or feces, hoarding, or rummaging through other's belongings.

- **Inappropriate public sexual behavior or public disrobing**

- **Resisting care** — examples include verbal or physical resistance to taking medications, taking injections, completing a variety of activities of daily living (ADLs), or eating.

The daily occurrence of such behaviors is disruptive to both the person and others with whom the person comes in contact. Such behaviors may lead to restricting the person's mobility or interactions with others, and in worst cases to functional decline. The immediate goal of care is to reduce the frequency to less than daily occurrences and eventually to eliminate all occurrences.

For those exhibiting these behaviors less than daily, the immediate goal of care is to prevent the behaviors from increasing in frequency and secondarily to eliminate them.

These behavior symptoms are most often set in motion by a declining cognitive status or episodes of severe mental illness, although they can have other causes as well. Thus, understanding the nature of the problem and addressing the underlying causes have the potential to improve the quality of the person's life and the quality of the lives of those with whom the person interacts.

Overall Goals of Care

- Eliminate underlying conditions or stressors that contribute to behavioral problems.

- Decrease the frequency or intensity of the behavior problems and prevent future escalation of the problems.

- Prevent secondary complications arising from the behaviors (for example, developing unsettled relationships with others, being abused by others, being physically restrained, or being admitted to a long-term care facility).

- Help staff and family caregivers cope with the existence of remaining behavior problems.

Behavior CAP Trigger

TRIGGERED TO REDUCE THE OCCURRENCE OF DAILY BEHAVIORS

This group includes persons who display any of the following behaviors (or their equivalent) daily:

- Wandering
- Verbally abusing others
- Physically abusing others
- Socially inappropriate or disruptive behavior
- Inappropriate public sexual behavior or public disrobing
- Resisting care

This triggered group includes about 10% of persons in long-term care facilities, 3% of persons receiving home care, and less than 1% of older adults living independently in the community. Over a 90-day period, about one-third of these persons will improve so that none of these behaviors are exhibited daily.

TRIGGERED TO PREVENT BEHAVIORS FROM OCCURRING DAILY

This group includes persons who exhibit any of the previously mentioned behaviors on a less than daily basis (or when frequency was not present on the assessment, the behavior tended to be easily altered).

This triggered group includes about 8% of persons in long-term care facilities, 7% of persons receiving home care, and less than 1% of older adults living independently in the community.

NOT TRIGGERED

This group includes persons who have not exhibited any of the previously mentioned behaviors in the observation period during the last 3 days.

This group accounts for about 82% of persons in long-term care facilities, 90% of persons receiving home care, and 99% of older adults living independently in the community. Appropriate care for these persons is limited to monitoring for any unexpected new problematic behaviors.

Behavior CAP Guidelines

Initial considerations. For persons displaying behavioral symptoms, a three-step approach to care is recommended.

- Step 1: Characterize the specific nature of the behavioral symptoms. Assume that the behaviors displayed may be a means for the person to communicate the presence of existing or new health problems, discomfort, or fears. To ignore this possibility can further isolate someone who has limited cognitive skills or severe mental health problems.

- Step 2: As best as possible, identify the factors causing or exacerbating the behavior. Often disruptive behaviors are new, and as such, the person may have modifiable problems that can be addressed through good quality care. The review that follows focuses on the principal causal factors that must be considered. When a specific cause is identified as the probable explanation, work with the physician, other care professionals, and when possible, the person, to establish a remedial plan of care.

- Step 3: Build on the person's strengths.

Step 1: Characterize the specific nature of the behavioral symptoms.

Active behaviors are often a form of communication, possibly about a mental or physical illness, an unmet need or fear, or the person's environment. Some are obvious, such as screaming or physical aggression. Other behaviors are less obvious, such as withdrawal from activities, isolation, or fear-induced agitation. In clarifying the nature of the behavior and related behavioral symptoms, consider the following:

- If the person is able to communicate, ask directly about his or her view of the situation. Does the person have an explanation for the behavior? Was he or she afraid? In pain? Excited or agitated? Hypervigilant? Was he or she aware of the consequences of the action?

- Describe the behavior in specific terms to facilitate understanding of its source or meaning, describing the behavior and what was happening when the behavior occurred.

  - Was aggressive behavior provoked (responsive) or unprovoked, especially when considered from the person's perspective?

  - Was it offensive (attacking someone else) or defensive (protecting oneself)?

  - Was it purposeful?

  - Was there an intent to harm in the behavior or was it a reflexive response?

  - Did it occur during specific activities (such as a bath)?

  - Was there any pattern, such as occurring at certain times of day?

  - Who was in the vicinity and involved?

- Did the environment influence the person's behavior (for example, lighting, noise, or setting)?

- Was it a reaction to a particular action, such as the person being physically moved?

- Is the person affected by sensory problems, particularly related to vision and hearing? If the person has problems with vision, is he or she often startled by others appearing in his or her field of vision unexpectedly? Does the person become confused by being unable to understand others because of hearing problems?

Step 2: Identify the factors causing or exacerbating the behavior.

Does the person have a long-standing mental health problem possibly associated with the behavioral disturbances? Examples include schizophrenia, bipolar disorder, depression, anxiety disorder, and post-traumatic stress disorder. A detailed psychiatric evaluation and a physician-directed plan of care are required when these conditions stand behind the disruptive behavior.

- Common symptoms include delusions, hallucinations, motor excitation, grandiosity, hostility, irritability, hyperarousal state, sleeplessness, flashbacks, startled responses, and phobias (for example, fear of needles, or fear of leaving the room).

- Some of these conditions can be addressed with medical or drug treatment. [See Mood CAP.] Others that are less responsive to traditional therapies should still be identified, understood, and addressed in care planning. For example, the physician may recommend a combination of drug interventions and nondrug interventions.

- Persons exhibiting long-standing problem behaviors related to psychiatric conditions may lack the ability to develop strategies to bring trouble in their lives under their own control. These persons may place others in danger of physical assault, intimidation, or embarrassment. They also place themselves at increased risk of being stigmatized, isolated, abused, and neglected by loved ones and those who provide care.

Does the person have dementia or recent cognitive loss? Examples include Alzheimer's disease, a stroke, and a decline in the person's Cognitive Performance Scale (CSP) score. [See Cognitive Loss CAP.]

- Did the symptoms occur suddenly, following a recent decline in the person's cognitive performance? In this instance, assume that an acute state of confusion or delirium is present. For people with a recognized dementia and existing behavior problems, delirium is often best identified when there is a rather sudden increase in frequency of the existing behavioral symptoms or the onset of new behavioral symptoms. When delirium is present, every effort must be made to identify and treat the underlying causes of the delirium. [See Delirium CAP.] The possible direct causes to be addressed include the onset of a new/acute illness, the reoccurrence of a chronic illness, or changes in medication regimen.

- Behavioral problems in dementia sometimes can be relieved by medications designed for dementia. Consider consulting the physician about these medications.

- Could the person be trying to communicate an unmet need? Does the person have difficulty making him- or herself understood? The person may be unable to communicate stress such as the urge to urinate, have an inability to know where to go, or experience pain on urination. Similarly, a person may display a challenging behavior because he or she does not recognize a caregiver or finds the environment unfamiliar and frightening.

- Does the person have other types of discomfort or needs that he or she cannot verbalize?

  - For example, is the person disrobing in public because the clothing is too tight or uncomfortable?

  - Is fatigue leading to lessened impulse control by the person?

  - Is the person wandering because he or she feels the urge to urinate but is too disoriented to find a bathroom?

  - A person partially paralyzed by a stroke may get frustrated, angry, and physically aggressive when caregivers do not understand his or her attempts to communicate.

  - A person with impaired mobility may need to be repositioned if he or she has been in the same position for a prolonged period of time.

- Is the person misinterpreting the environment or actions of others?

  - A person with memory loss may forget that he or she is married or make inappropriate advances to a member of the opposite sex.

  - Similarly, a person with Alzheimer's disease, seeing a housekeeper straightening up the room and picking up clothing, may interpret the unfamiliar person as a thief.

  - In such cases, agitation, verbal abusiveness, resistance to care, or even physical aggression may occur.

■ Can the behaviors of the cognitively impaired person be tolerated? For many persons with chronic progressive dementia, certain behaviors may continue despite remedial treatments or interventions. Occasionally, the behaviors will be distressing, yet often can be accommodated.

　■ For example, many persons who wander can be accommodated without restraints in a hazard-free environment.

　■ Similarly, if the needs and patterns of persons with repetitive behaviors or catastrophic reactions are anticipated, care plan strategies may be developed and followed to avoid escalation of the behavior. For example, if the person becomes agitated and is known to strike out at staff during ADL care, stopping the activity at the first sign of agitation, and trying later, may prevent the striking out.

Does the person have a new or acute physical health problem or a flare-up of a known chronic condition that may be causing or aggravating a behavior symptom?

■ Conditions such as delirium, an infection, dehydration, constipation, and congestive heart failure are physical health problems that can cause behavior disturbances. [A review of the Delirium, Dehydration, and Undernutrition CAPs is warranted.]

■ Determine if anything interferes with the person's ability to get enough sleep (for example, light, noise, frequent vital sign checks during the night, or a roommate with different sleep patterns).

■ Is the person in pain? This can result in depression, reduced mobility, social isolation, sleep disruption, and behavioral outbursts. The person may be startled if touched or moved in a way that aggravates the pain. If the person is receiving a pain medication or another pain management therapy, review it to find out whether it is being administered regularly and whether the dosage or intervention is enough to manage the pain without breakthrough pain. [See Pain CAP.]

Could the onset or aggravation of problem behaviors be associated with medication side effects?

■ Is the person receiving a new medication or has there been a change in dosage? Review the length of time from the change to the onset or worsening of behavioral symptoms.

■ Is the person receiving any medication known to contribute to or aggravate behaviors? Common medications causing side effects leading to behavior problems include:

　■ Antiparkinsonian drugs can cause hypersexuality and socially inappropriate behavior, such as public masturbation or unsought sexual advances.

　■ Some medications, such as sedatives, centrally active antihypertensives, some cardiac drugs, and anticholinergic agents can cause paranoid delusions, induce delirium symptoms, or cause reversible cognitive damage.

　■ Bronchodilators or other drugs used to treat respiratory problems, such as chronic obstructive pulmonary disease (COPD) or asthma, can increase agitation and cause difficulty sleeping. Too much caffeine and nicotine can also have a similar adverse side effect.

　■ Many medications and substances can impair impulse control. Examples include benzodiazepines, sedatives, alcohol, or any product containing alcohol (for example, some cough medicines).

Do family members and caregivers interact appropriately with the person?
The actions and responses of family members and caregivers can aggravate or even cause behavioral outbursts.

- Do caregivers or family members have unrealistic expectations for what the person can do, considering the person's physical and cognitive function?

  - If appropriate, are caregivers dividing larger tasks (such as dressing) into a string of smaller activities the person can perform?

  - Are family members and formal caregivers aware of the person's cognitive patterns and physical functioning?

  - Do family members or caregivers express frustration with the person?

- Do family members and caregivers provide cues, reminders, and reassurance to help the person make sense of things?

- Are family members and caregivers asking too many questions or making too many statements at once? A person with communication problems—either physical or cognitive—could become frustrated coping with the information provided.

- Are there major unresolved sources of interpersonal conflict between the person and family members, other care recipients, or staff? Previous life events or dysfunctional patterns in social relationships may be an underlying cause of current behavior problems.

Is a behavior management program in place? What are the key elements of the program? Review how the person has previously responded to attempts to change or alter the behavior. What was tried? How well did it work?

- Is there a scheduled, at least monthly, drug regime review program involving nurses, physicians, and the pharmacist? Evaluate whether there is congruence between psychiatric diagnoses and the prescription of psychotropic drugs. Assess whether there is a need to increase the use of a drug or whether it can be tapered off.

- Is there a documented behavior management program in place? Does it reference how others can best approach the person so that he or she reacts appropriately? Is there a strategy for increasing staff interactions with the person? Have staff received specific instructions on how to carry out such exchanges? Are they encouraged to enter into such exchanges, and is there a process for documenting the results? Does the program include specific behavioral therapy sessions led by a trained leader? Does it include structural activities? Has there been an environmental review, and have steps been taken to alter problematic stimuli?

- Has the program set specific improvement targets, either by changes in type of behavior, frequency of behavior, or date of expected change? Have specific changes been documented?

- Does the program serving the person have access to mental health specialists for evaluations? Has the person had a mental health evaluation, if needed?

- Evaluate the benefits for continuing interventions by determining whether or not the person's behavior improved over the last 90 days.

- Consider what other less restrictive approaches might be used if the current intervention is stopped.

- Track the person's response to a decrease or change in existing interventions, particularly changes in the use of psychotropic medications or restraints. Use of physical restraints should be considered a last resort option, if used at all.

Step 3: Build on the person's strengths.

The care plan should include strategies for improving the person's quality of life by enhancing his or her personal, social, and environmental strengths. Consider areas of strength that have been evident over the person's life in addition to those that are present today. Increase the opportunities for the person to draw on his or her strengths in daily life.

- When is the person comfortable and relaxed (for example, time of day, location, type of activity, social environment)? Are there factors present in these circumstances that can be used to reduce instances of problem behaviors?

- Which family members or caregivers are able to engage in calm, composed interactions with the person? Speak with these individuals to learn what they find to be effective in engaging the person in activities without agitation.

- What is important to the person now? What was important to the person previously? Does the person have opportunities to engage in activities that he or she values? Are there objects of sentimental value to the person, and does he or she have access to those objects (for example, photographs of family members, cards)?

  - Be aware of cultural factors that may be a central part of the person's identity. Are there events that have been important for the person to celebrate? What can be done to support interactions with the person's cultural community?

- Where is the person most relaxed? What features of the physical and social environment are associated with positive behavior patterns? Does the person demonstrate less agitated behavior in quiet settings, less crowded environments, or environments with reduced visual stimuli?

Additional Resources

Fogel B. 1997. Behavioral symptoms. In Morris JN, Lipsitz LA, Murphy KM, Belleville-Taylor P, eds. *Quality care in the nursing home.* St. Louis, MO: Mosby.

Gwyther LP. 2001. Caring for persons with Alzheimer's disease: A manual for facility staff. Washington, DC: American Health Care Association and the Alzheimer's Association. Alzheimer's Association: www.alz.org

Hirdes JP, Fries BE, Rabinowitz T, Morris JN. 2007. Comprehensive assessment of persons with bipolar disorder in long-term care settings: The potential of the interRAI family of instruments. In Sajatovic M, Blow FC, eds. *Bipolar disorders in late life.* Baltimore, MD: Johns Hopkins University Press.

Mace NL, Rabins PV. 2000. The 36-hour a day family guide to caring for persons with Alzheimer's disease, related dementing illnesses, and memory loss in later life. Baltimore, MD: Johns Hopkins University Press.

Robinson A, Spencer B, White LA. 1999. Understanding difficult behaviors: Some practical suggestions for coping with Alzheimer's disease and related illnesses. Geriatric Education Center of Michigan, Ypsilanti, MI.

Authors

Catherine Hawes, PhD
John P. Hirdes, PhD
John N. Morris, PhD, MSW

Abusive Relationship CAP

Problem

The Abusive Relationship CAP is designed to identify persons who are in situations of potential abuse or neglect, and to aid in the decisions for action. In some countries and communities, reporting such cases to a designated agency is mandated.

Mistreatment may be an act of commission (abuse) or omission (neglect). While in some instances it may be an intentional conscious attempt to inflict suffering, it may also be an unintentional act, a result of inadequate knowledge, infirmity, depression, burnout, or inattentiveness on the part of the caregiver.

The expressions of mistreatment can be grouped under four main headings:

- **Physical abuse** — Inflicting physical pain or injury, including sexual molestation.

- **Psychological abuse** — Inflicting mental anguish, including humiliation and intimidation.

- **Neglect** — Failure to fulfill a caregiving duty, including, for example, the denial of food, health related services, or abandonment.

- **Financial abuse** — The improper or illegal use of funds and assets.

It is imperative to respond to evidence of abuse. Persons who experience abuse may be at immediate risk of injury or other serious health problems. In addition, abuse affects other aspects of life, including psychological well-being, social participation, and community involvement. An ongoing concern, even after abuse has ceased, is the risk of post-traumatic stress disorder, which may include serious psychiatric symptoms such as severe depression and recurrence of suicidal ideation (suicidality).

Overall Goals of Care

- Evaluate the capacity of the person to decide about his or her own welfare, and to have an understanding of the consequences of those decisions.

- Determine the level of risk to the person.

- Determine the need for immediate interventions, such as social services, medical care, court orders for protection, or relocation of the person.

- Monitor for long-term mental health consequences related to abuse.

Abusive Relationship CAP Trigger

This CAP identifies persons of all ages who are in situations of neglect or abuse, or who are at substantial risk of either. The short-term goal is to decide whether the situation requires immediate action, while the medium- to long-term goal is to manage psychosocial consequences arising from a history of abuse. Research suggests that about one-third of the persons who trigger this CAP will no longer trigger it 90 days later. However, there is a persistent risk over the life course of depression, anxiety, and impaired social function if the psychological consequences of abuse are not addressed effectively.

TRIGGERED — HIGHEST RISK STATUS

This subgroup includes persons who meet both of the following criteria:

- **One or more** of the following direct indicators of abuse are present:
  - Fearful of a family member, caregiver, or close acquaintance
  - Unusually poor hygiene, unkempt or disheveled appearance
  - Neglected, abused, or mistreated
- **Two or more** of the following "stressors" are present:
  - Depression — Depression Rating Scale score of 3 or higher
  - Poor nutrition — includes any of following: substantial recent weight loss, malnutrition, the consumption of one or fewer meals a day, insufficient fluid intake, body mass index of less than 19, or a decrease in food eaten
  - Anger or conflict with family or friends
  - Health issues — not in full compliance with medication regimen, medically unstable, or self-rated health is poor
  - Residential setting judged to be unable to meet needs and it would be best if the person moved
  - Caregiver is distressed, angry, or depressed
  - Social isolation — withdrawal from activities, reduced social interaction, or expression of loneliness

About 2 to 6% of persons (of all ages) receiving home care and less than 1% of older adults living independently in the community will be triggered in the "Highest Risk Status."

TRIGGERED — MODERATE RISK STATUS

This subgroup includes persons who meet only the first of the two above criteria; that is, they have one or more of the direct indicators of abuse and do not have two or more stressors.

About 1 to 6% of persons receiving home care and less than 1% of older adults living independently in the community will be triggered in the "Moderate Risk Status."

NOT TRIGGERED

This group includes all other persons.

Abusive Relationship CAP Guidelines

Is the behavior abusive? In determining whether a behavior is abusive, neglectful, or exploitive, the frequency, duration, severity, and likely consequences of the observations should be assessed. In addition, both the objective circumstances surrounding the behavior and the person's view of the situation should be considered. Does he or she see it as abusive? Is he or she receptive to a corrective course of action? Are there cultural factors that result in acceptance of the behavior or that make the person less willing to respond?

- **For the "Highest Risk Status" subgroup** there is a high likelihood of the presence of abuse with imminent physical or mental health concerns. For these persons, consider the following factors:

  - Is there a history of violence, abuse, neglect, or exploitation by the caregiver, including physical abuse of others?

  - Are formal services being provided at an adequate, reliable level?

  - Are agency staff aware of the issue and have steps been taken to address the recognized problems?

  - Should the person be removed from the abusive environment immediately?

  - Does the caregiver and family understand the abuse and are they willing to try to correct the problems?

  - Is substance abuse an issue for the person or for the caregiver?

  - Are there immediate mental health concerns that place the person at risk of harm to self or others?

- **For the "Moderate Risk Status" subgroup**, you should screen further for possible abuse and neglect. While abuse or neglect may be suspected, this may not always be true. There are a variety of reasons why initial indicators of abuse are in fact explained by other factors. For example, the caregiver (or others) may be falsely accused of abuse because of mental health problems experienced by the person. Sometimes a person with cognitive impairment may not recall the benign cause of a bruise. In evaluating potential abuse without supporting indicators, alternative explanations should be considered. However, the assessment of the situation should be as thorough as possible to ensure that cases of actual abuse are not inadvertently discounted. Particular attention should be given to

  - The immediate and long-term context of the presenting problem (for example, is there a family history of abuse?)

  - The risk of abuse, neglect, or exploitation (for example, how vulnerable is the person, and are there clear power inequalities between the person and the caregiver?)

  - The severity and frequency of the problem

  - The immediacy of the risk (for example, what is the likelihood of immediate harm to the person in the present environment?)

  - The caregiver's perspective (for example, does the caregiver feel that he or she is part of the problem?)

  - Cultural factors that may be barriers to identifying or responding to abuse

Interview the person in a nonthreatening manner. The discussion should occur with the person alone (not in the presence of the alleged or possible abuser), although at first it may not be possible to do so. The person's confirmation of the mistreatment is an important factor in deciding the nature of further action. Ask the person to describe his or her feelings about the abusive event(s). Does the person describe the event(s) as inducing an intense feeling of fear or horror? What is the person's response to other severe life events? When the person denies mistreatment, you must make a decision about its validity.

Investigate the potential abuse. To decide if abuse is present, it may be advisable to obtain information from health or social service professionals, relatives, and service providers. An interview with the individual suspected of being abusive (if appropriate) can be helpful in developing a successful intervention strategy. Explain to the caregiver that part of the regular interview process is talking to the caregiver separately from the person. When doing this, evaluate the goodwill, health, mental and emotional status, and competency of the caregiver.

It may be difficult to assess the extent of financial abuse in the absence of detailed information on financial resources, spending patterns, and cultural and family norms. Although the need to make difficult economic tradeoffs (for example, among health care, prescribed medications, heating, food) may occur with some cases of financial abuse, not all economic tradeoffs are due to abuse and not all persons who are financially abused are forced to make economic tradeoffs.

Treatment. The response to abuse, neglect, or exploitation will vary according to individual cases, the severity of the abuse or its potential, and the laws of a jurisdiction. Often social service agencies can work with a caregiver to lessen or mitigate factors that contribute to possible abuse or neglect. Homemaking services and respite care can help in allowing the caregiver time away from the person.

The stressors referenced for those at highest risk are all highly prevalent problems. Many have associated CAPs that should be considered.

- About two-thirds of those triggered will have health problems, including ADL and cognitive impairment.

- One-half will have problems in the areas of social isolation, depression, anxiety, loss of pleasure in life (anhedonia), and anger or conflict with family.

- About 30% will have poor nutrition, identified to be in need of relocation, or have informal caregivers who are distressed, angry, or depressed.

Relevant Clinical Assessment Protocols to be considered to assist in resolving these problems include Social Relationship, Activities, Informal Support, Mood, Behavior, Dehydration, Cognitive Loss, and Undernutrition.

In constructing a plan of care, the following issues should be addressed:

- Is the person in immediate physical danger? If so, immediate action must be taken to address the problems. This might include steps to immediately remove the person from the present environment. Consider the potential reaction of the abusive individual and how he or she may respond to this move, as well as that of the person being abused.

- Will the person accept the intervention?

- Does the abusive individual acknowledge his or her role and will he or she accept entry into a therapeutic program?

- Will providing (more) formal direct care services lead to an improvement in the situation?

- Would the caregiver benefit from counseling or medical treatment to help bear the present burden?

- If the allegations of abuse appear to be unsubstantiated, would the person benefit from counseling or psychiatric assessment and treatment?

- Is the person showing indications of post-traumatic stress in relation to the abuse? If so, it may be necessary to make a referral for appropriate psychiatric care.

Follow-up and monitoring. Periodic reassessment is needed in all cases, especially when the evidence of abuse is inconclusive. Even if a person refuses help, it may still be beneficial to provide written information about emergency assistance numbers and suitable referrals.

For persons who have had the Abusive Relationships CAP triggered in a previous assessment, it is important to monitor for signs of mental health problems even if the CAP is no longer triggered. There might be new information available that will help assure the presence or absence of abuse. In addition, conditions that were antecedents or precipitating factors in prior episodes of abuse should be observed for and addressed if their recurrence is noted.

Additional Resources

Clearinghouse on Abuse and Neglect of the Elderly (CANE): www.cane.udel.edu
Ontario Network for the Prevention of Elder Abuse: www.onpea.org

---

Authors

John N. Morris, PhD, MSW
John P. Hirdes, PhD

Part III

Social Life CAPs

Activities CAP

Problem

The Activities CAP identifies persons with some cognitive reserve who have either withdrawn from activities or who are uneasy entering into activities and social relationships. The goal of care is to identify strategies for helping these persons increase their activity involvement (for example, playing cards, reading books, reminiscing, or watching movies).

An active lifestyle, especially one within the constraints of a person's functional capacity and prior engagement patterns, can be essential to the maintenance of a positive outlook and an overall sense of self-esteem and well-being. About two-thirds of those triggered in this CAP will neither have a consistent positive outlook nor find meaning in day-to-day life.

From this perspective, it is important to reach out to these persons. We need to recognize also that their general functional and cognitive profile will not diverge significantly from other persons in their living environments. Thus, the crucial task is not to address other complicating problems, but rather to proceed directly to attempts to better engage the person in a variety of leisure activities. At the same time, the activity programs offered should be tailored to the cognitive, physical, and social abilities of the person.

It is important to ensure that planning considers the preferred activities of the person, regardless of whether they are passive or active, and not the biases of the caregiver. These activities should focus on helping the person fulfill his or her wishes, use his or her physical and cognitive skills, provide enjoyment, and provide an avenue to interact with others.

Overall Goals of Care

- Talk with the person to identify why the person has withdrawn from activities or is ill at ease in joining with others.

- When present, address functional, medical, or psychological causes that affect the person's ability to participate in activities.

- Identify methods of increasing activity, while keeping in mind the person's usual preferred level of involvement.

- Give the person an opportunity to succeed.

Activities CAP Trigger

TRIGGERED
This subgroup is defined by the presence of **all three** of the following factors:

- First, the person's involvement level in activities is less than most of time;

- Second, the person has some ability to engage in everyday decision making (Independent to Moderately Impaired in Cognitive Skills for Daily Decision Making); and

- Third, two or more of the following are present:

  - Withdrawn from activities of interest

  - Reduced social interaction

  - Not at ease interacting with others

  - Not at ease doing planned or structured activities

  - Not at ease doing self-initiated activities

This subgroup includes about 25% of persons in long-term care facilities.

NOT TRIGGERED
All other persons. The "Not Triggered" subgroup includes about 75% of persons in long-term care facilities.

Activities CAP Guidelines

Approach to the Person with Problems Related to Activities

Initial assessment. Does the person have discrete activity preferences? To answer this question one must talk with the person and/or a knowledgeable family member or friend (when they visit — and remember that about 80% of these persons will maintain strong relations with family).

- What were the person's activity preferences prior to coming into the program?

  - Were they passive or active? (For example, did the person spend large amounts of time watching television or reading?)

  - Did they involve activities, with or without family, outside of the home (for example, church, clubs, sporting events, travel, dining)?

  - Were they centered almost entirely on family — spouse, children, and grandchildren?

  - Were they centered almost entirely on nonfamily/community service support?

- In what activities is the person currently involved?

  - Create a comprehensive list of leisure pursuits, including those done alone and/or self-directed and those done with others and/or planned by others.

  - Do visitors come to see the person and, if so, what kinds of activities do they pursue together?

  - What scheduled programs does the person participate in at the time of the assessment?

  - Does participation in programs fluctuate with seasonal program changes or are there patterns of change apparent in the person's activity involvement?

- In what types of other activities would the person have an interest in participating? Include those that are not currently available or offered to the person.

- What unique skills or knowledge does the person have that he or she could pass on to others? Does he or she know how to play bridge or chess? Can he or she help others deal with complex forms (for example, tax forms)? Is he or she knowledgeable about a topic that others might also have an interest in (for example, baseball)?

Determination of the nature of problems that reduce participation.

- When determining activity needs or potential interventions for care planning purposes, it is important to determine "why" a person chooses to participate or not participate in leisure pursuits.

  - Does the person hold back because of functional or cognitive reasons? Look at issues of stamina, mobility, balance, ability to express self, ability to understand others, and ability to make decisions.

  - Consider psychosocial well-being indicators, such as initiative and social involvement.

  - Has the person been made to feel unwelcome? Do those already involved in an activity draw boundaries that are difficult to cross?

  - Does the person's health condition represent a barrier? Is the person incontinent, or is pain an issue?

  - Is the person hindered because of embarrassment or unease due to the presence of health-related equipment (for example, tubes, oxygen tank, colostomy bag, or wheelchair)?

  - Does the person have a lack of resources to engage in the activity?

  - Are there opportunities for the person to get to know others in the living environment (for example, shared dining, afternoon drinks, monthly birthday parties, reminiscence groups)?

  - Do cultural expectations lessen the person's interest in the available activities?

  - Has the person always been uneasy in joining with others? If so, would reaching out to the person succeed (and has it in the past) or is the person just someone who requires more passive or self-directed activities?

- Is it an issue of activity availability?

  - The facility in which one lives may not have an organized program in areas that the person finds interesting — games, exercise, religious discussion.

  - Is it possible to make participation in an activity less demanding, thereby facilitating the person's participation in the activity?

  - Does the person have sufficient private time for independent and self-directed pursuits?

- Are there environmental or staffing issues that hinder participation?

  - Are there physical barriers that prevent the person from gaining access to the space in which the activity is held?

  - Does the facility have enough specific staff responsible for social activities?

  - Does staff lack time to involve others in current activity programs?

  - Does staff intimidate the person, failing to recognize the fragile nature of the person?

Treatment and monitoring. The plan to deal with inactivity and re-involvement must be tailored to the person's strengths and preferences. Activities that are too challenging may exclude the person with more severe impairments, and activities that are insufficiently challenging may not be motivating to the person. Activities programs can be used to support a variety of purposes, including rehabilitation or restoration of functioning, prevention or decline, or simply increased participation. In addition to offering activity programs, it is important to recognize that leisure education should be considered as part of a comprehensive strategy to reduce inactivity. For some persons it will be important that the treatment program include education and counseling on how to incorporate leisure into the person's life, whether at home or in the long-term care facility setting. Interventions that incorporate the family into the person's leisure activities may be particularly beneficial.

- Passive and self-directed leisure activities may be the most immediate avenues to re-engage the person. About 90% of these persons would be comfortable with activities that take place in his or her own room. Among activities that would be of interest to many of those triggered are watching television, listening to music, and talking one-on-one with another person. To a somewhat lesser extent, about 40% of those triggered are interested in reading.

- Although there is cultural variation in the triggered group, a significant percentage identified a preference for the following social, interactive activities: spiritually related activity (50%), playing cards (40%), and involvement in a craft (25%).

- Among the physical activities of interest are exercise (about 45%) and walking outdoors (50%).

- Tailor activities programs to the person's strengths and preferences.

  - Consider whether available activity options are age appropriate and culturally appropriate for the person.

  - Would it benefit the person to extend his or her leisure pursuits to include others that may have similar interests?

  - Avoid activities that the person would find embarrassing, demeaning, or uncomfortable. Be careful to recognize that such reactions are affected by both individual personality traits and sociocultural factors.

  - Identify activities that may be interesting and challenging to the person but do not clearly exceed his or her cognitive or physical abilities.

- Be attentive to signs of psychiatric conditions. If the person has a Depression Rating Scale (DRS) score of 3 or more, bring it to the attention of a mental health professional. This may be an indication of the presence of depression and will require appropriate intervention.

- Symptoms such as withdrawal from social activities and reduced social interaction can be the result of mental health problems such as depression or schizophrenia.

- Pervasive conflict with other persons, family, or staff can create a serious barrier to participation in and enjoyment of activities programs. Identify ways to support conflict resolution if it appears to be prolonged.

- Find ways to involve family, friends, community groups, and volunteers. Discuss visiting patterns with family.

Additional Resources

Mace N, Perschbacher R, Tuplin H, Westerman M, Carlson J, Schober G. 1997. Activities programming. In Morris JN, Lipsitz LA, Murphy KM, Belleville-Taylor P, eds. *Quality care in the nursing home.* St. Louis, MO: Mosby. **Note:** This chapter provides an overview of the problem and a detailed approach to clinical assessment, dealing with obstacles and challenges, and tips for care planning.

McPherson BD. 1998. Studying aging processes: Theory and research. In *Aging as a social process.* New York: Harcourt Brace & Company.

Therapeutic Recreation Directory: www.recreationtherapy.com is a useful Web site that provides numerous suggestions for activity programs, relevant publications, and links to other related Web sites.

Authors

John P. Hirdes, PhD

John N. Morris, PhD, MSW

Informal Support CAP

Problem

The Informal Support CAP looks to situations where a person will need the help of others, seeking to identify situations where agencies or companies may have to step in to provide help. In these situations, the needs of the person usually exceed the response capabilities of the informal care network. Informal care reflects instrumental and personal support provided to the person by family, friends, and neighbors. Instrumental support (IADL) includes meal preparation, housework, managing finances, and so on. Personal support (ADL) includes mobility in bed, dressing, toilet use, and so on.

On any given day, independent adults will spend a certain amount of time performing instrumental activities, such as tidying up the residence and cooking, as well as carrying out personal activities of daily living, such as bathing, grooming, and dressing. They typically perform all or almost all instrumental and personal activities of daily living on their own. The principal exception is persons living with others, where some of the tasks of daily life may be shared or performed by others in the household.

Nevertheless, with aging, as chronic diseases and disabilities increase, instrumental activities are usually the first areas in which a loss of partial or full personal self-sufficiency can be expected. As that loss occurs, family members and friends typically step forward to help the person carry out these tasks, including help with meals, shopping, and transportation. Alternatively, when there is a close personal relationship with a paid domestic helper, that person may assume additional responsibilities. The total time needed to carry out these activities will remain about what it was before, only now the person performs less of the activity, with that time replaced by family and friends performing more. Such increases in informal support seldom tear at the bonds that tie the person to the family. Love and a sense of duty drive the family to step forward. The process is usually natural and unspoken, with family simply stepping in to do what is necessary. The person is seldom left in a dangerous or untenable situation, and as a new need arises, family and friends almost always step forward to pick up all or most of the slack.

Overall Goals of Care

- Identify families who cannot provide informal care that will fully compensate for the care needs of persons with a decline in IADL and ADL, and develop a family-agency plan to meet the needs of the person.

- Identify persons with no primary informal caregiver and consider formal care services intervention.

- Identify persons whose problems may improve and thus whose needs may decrease, and assist the family to step forward on a short-term basis.

In this CAP, however, we seek to identify persons whose informal support systems may be at a higher risk of not fully responding to their unfolding needs. What distinguishes these persons is that when first seen they are likely to be receiving lower levels of informal help, irrespective of their functional disability level.

This CAP does not seek to isolate informal helpers having stress or strain, for this factor by itself is not crucial to the level of informal care provided to the person. Informal helpers usually continue to provide help even when stress and strain are present.

Informal Support CAP Trigger

This CAP trigger identifies persons who currently require help with instrumental activities of daily living, focusing on those who have families that are challenged to respond fully to the emerging needs of the person. While the family members will almost always be sympathetic to the needs of the person, formal agencies need to prepare to step in to provide higher levels of formal support services to such persons. Where formal agencies are not yet involved, family members must be encouraged to reach out for help.

This CAP is not designed to assign blame or make a judgment on a particular person's informal care network. Rather, it seeks to identify persons who have an informal support network that will benefit from having a "back-up" plan or alternative arrangement in place as the person declines over time. Informal support systems in situations such as this are called "brittle."

TRIGGERED IF BOTH OF THE FOLLOWING ARE TRUE

- Not independent (setup help permitted) in one or more of the following IADL difficulty (capacity to perform) areas: meals, housework, shopping, and transportation.

- Two or more of the following apply:

  - Alone for long periods of time or all of the time during the day

  - Lives alone or in a group setting with nonrelatives

  - No primary informal helper present

For those in the community, every point of decline in IADL capacity translates into about a 10% loss of personal self-sufficiency in instrumental activities. The triggered group includes about 40% of persons receiving home care and 10% of older adults living independently in the community.

For this triggered group, informal replacement levels are less than one-half of the levels of those not triggered. However, should there be a change in the factors comprising the trigger (for example, no longer lives alone), the informal support system responsiveness will change. Nevertheless, for those triggered, the person is likely to find him- or herself having to continue to carry out a higher proportion of instrumental activities. This can challenge the person and result in these functional activities being less well performed.

In a home care environment, the goal would be to identify where there is a gap in family response potential, and to provide a formal maintenance service whenever possible. When such service is provided, the person will receive help in completing activities that exceed his or her functional abilities.

NOT TRIGGERED   All other persons.

Check for declines in IADLs and ADLs, establish care needs, and identify families who cannot provide informal care that will fully compensate. A discussion with the family (or the person) should take place to determine the nature of the difficulties being faced and explore available alternatives such as the following:

- Help the person move in with a loved one; the agency could consider moving support.

- Draw up a joint family-agency plan for meeting the needs of the person. To create such a plan often requires that the person is eligible for formal services and that there is a payment mechanism in place to provide the needed level of services. Where this has not been determined, a formal application for service coverage will need to be made.

- If access to more intensive formal care is not an option, efforts should be made to assist the family members to explore areas where they might be able to do more. In addition, a review of the other CAPs may help to identify whether there is a possibility for the person to improve. If the answer is "yes," this may be helpful information for the family to be aware of because the increase in help can then be seen as a temporary measure. If the answer is "no," the need to provide more prolonged support should be anticipated.

- Some family members may be strained or burdened; relieving these conditions could make them willing or able to do more for the person. As a first step, review the Abusive Relationship CAP; if abuse is present, it must be addressed first. Assuming this is not the case, consider the following:

  - Would respite care for the person provide an opportunity for family members to improve their health or relieve their strain?

  - Are the family members misinformed of the person's status? Should family contact levels be increased? Should family members in contact with the person keep other potential helpers "in the loop"?

  - Do family members have the capacity to purchase services to help the person?

  - Has the person refused offers of help? Some persons will refuse efforts to address their needs, whether from informal or formal sources. Often, in such situations, the person has a history of refusing help, and all the assessor or the family can do is provide oversight and wait for a suitable time to offer informed counseling.

  - Family members may be concerned about taking on more than they can handle, and a simple educational exchange may help to counter their fears about the extent to which the person will continue to decline in the immediate future.

  - The primary caregiver needs specialized instruction and interim oversight on specialized care tasks (for example, how to deal effectively with new personal care needs, giving injections, or addressing emerging behavior problems).

  - Direct counseling and enrollment in support groups may provide family members with effective strategies to manage the stress and feelings of burden. It may be helpful to inform the family about resources available to them in the community such as Alzheimer's family support groups or mental health agencies.

  - Caregivers of such persons who are experiencing feelings of severe stress and burden may even decrease their informal care if these problems are not addressed.

No primary informal caregiver is present. The 15% of persons triggered with no primary informal caregiver receive the least amount of informal care. For persons in this group, 50% are widowed, 22% never married, and 17% are divorced. Most (80%) live in private homes or apartments. As these persons' health declines, they experience an increase in informal care similar to the persons triggered in the other groups, but at a lower level than the group not triggered.

■ For persons with no primary informal caregiver, who are receiving some informal help (for example, a grandniece calls once a week), the agency should explore the options listed in the previous section.

■ For persons with no primary informal caregiver who are receiving no informal care at all, formal care services need to be considered. As stated in the previous section, some persons consistently refuse formal and informal help. At times, the remaining course of action is to provide limited oversight and wait for a better time to offer informed counseling.

Review other triggered CAPs for areas in which the person might improve and thus need less help in the future. If such changes are possible and likely, the family may be more willing to step forward in the short term as the level of need by the person for long-term formal care can be expected to decrease as the person becomes more self-sufficient.

■ CAPs of special relevance include IADL CAP, ADL CAP, Cognitive Loss CAP, Prevention CAP, Behavior CAP, Mood CAP, and Delirium CAP.

Authors

John N. Morris, PhD, MSW
Naoki Ikegami, MD
John P. Hirdes, PhD
Jean-Claude Henrard, MD
Pauline Belleville-Taylor, RN, MS, CS

Social Relationship CAP

Problem

Involvement in social relationships is a vital aspect of life, with most adults having meaningful relationships with family, friends, and neighbors. When these relationships are challenged, a sense of distress often clouds other aspects of life. Decreases in a person's social relationships may affect psychological well-being and have an impact on mood, behavior, and physical activity. Conversely, declines in physical functioning or cognition, or a new onset or worsening of pain or other health problems, may affect both social relationships and mood. This may also be the case when one moves or has experienced the death of a loved one.

Many persons who are lonely are also depressed, and it can be difficult to know which came first, but for this CAP, the crucial consideration is that both must be treated together. For example, depression can be associated with irritability and anger leading to conflict in interpersonal relationships. Good social relationships can play an important role in buffering the negative effects of stress.

The Social Relationship CAP identifies factors associated with reduced social relationships and addresses interventions to facilitate social engagement. The initial interventions for this CAP thus focus on social re-engagement, mood, and behavior manifestations. But, one must also consider other contributing factors, such as mental health problems and poor health.

15

Overall Goals of Care

- Seek ways to engage the person with others (including caregivers).

- Identify and address any serious conflicts the person has with members of his or her support network.

- Identify underlying mental health problems that exacerbate interpersonal conflicts or contribute to the person's withdrawal from social activities.

- Identify methods of increasing a person's engagement in social activities, while keeping in mind the person's usual and preferred level of involvement.

- Treat underlying depression. [See Mood CAP.]

Social Relationship CAP Trigger

TRIGGERED FOR CARE PLAN FOLLOW-UP IF ALL THREE OF THE FOLLOWING ARE PRESENT

- Feels lonely (or either fails to pursue involvement in life of the facility or is distressed by declining social activity and the person is alone for long periods of time)*

- Has a reasonable level of cognitive assets (as indicated by a Cognitive Performance Scale score of 3 or lower)

- Has at least some ability to understand others (as indicated by having an Ability to Understand Others score that is less that the most severe — not "Rarely/Never Understands")

This group includes about 35% of persons in long-term care facilities, 15% of persons receiving home care, and 15% of older adults living independently in the community.

NOT TRIGGERED   All other persons. This group includes about 65% of persons in long-term care facilities, 85% of persons receiving home care, and 85% of older adults living independently in the community.

Social Relationship CAP Guidelines

Overview of Approach to Thinking about Social Relationships

Determine lifetime relationship patterns.

- Assess whether the person is lonely.

- Assess if loneliness is of recent onset. For some persons, low involvement in social relationships is consistent with a lifelong pattern of social engagement. For others, recent declines in social involvement, and associated loneliness, can be a sign of acute health complications and depression.

- When the assessment instrument does not include these questions, assess the following:

  - Person says or indicates he or she feels lonely.

  - Person feels distressed because of decline in social activities.

  - Over the past few years, there has been an absence of daily exchanges with relatives and friends.

Determine the nature of factors that may impinge on social exchanges.

- Health status factors:

  - ADL or IADL decline, especially in locomotion.

  - Health problem (for example, falls, pain, fatigue).

  - Mood and behavior problems. Some mental health problems may manifest themselves in various ways that have a direct impact on interpersonal relationships, or may arise because of the lack of contact with others. Withdrawal from activities of interest and reduced social interactions can be symptoms of mental health problems.

*This parenthetical criteria applies when the loneliness item is not available on the instrument.

- Changes in communication, vision, or cognition.
- Environmental factors:
  - Change in residence can lead to a loss of autonomy and reduced self-esteem.
  - Recent change in family situation or social network (for example, death of a close family member or friend).
  - No one in the person's living environment can be involved in daily informal exchanges with him or her.
- Medications may have side effects that can interfere with social interactions.

Supplemental Clinical Observations

Are changes in the person's patterns of social interaction only temporary fluctuations or are they more persistent in nature?

- Are the conflicts with others new or do they reflect persistent patterns?
- Does the person have a long-standing difficulty in adjusting to new situations?
- Does the person no longer take pleasure in activities that were previously important?
- How frequently did he or she participate in activities with others prior to the onset of a recent illness or functional decline?
- Does the person make statements indicating distress over how his or her life has changed?
- Do family or friends feel the person has changed in the way he or she relates to others?

Has the person demonstrated strengths in psychosocial functioning?

- Are there activities in which the person appears especially at ease in interacting with others?
- Are there other individuals who seem to bring out a more positive, optimistic side of the person?
- What positive traits distinguished the person as an individual prior to his or her illness?
- What gave the person a sense of satisfaction earlier in his or her life?

Does the person have a mental health or psychiatric condition that could affect social exchanges?

- Does the person have a diagnosis of depression, bipolar disorder, anxiety disorder, schizophrenia, or a personality disorder?
- Calculate the MDS Depression Rating Scale (DRS). A score of 3 or more indicates potential depression. [See Mood CAP.]
- Does the person use antipsychotic or antidepressant medications?
- Does the person feel stigmatized by taking psychiatric medications or having a mental health diagnosis?
- Do medication side effects impede social interactions?
- Does the person have increasing frequency of disturbing behaviors? [See Behavior CAP.]

- Is the person preoccupied with the past in a way that makes him or her unwilling or unable to respond to present social needs?

- Has there been a decline in cognitive functioning over the last 90 to 180 days? Use the MDS Cognitive Performance Scale (CPS) to evaluate the severity of the person's cognitive impairment, if any.

Are there situational factors that may impede the ability to interact with others?

- Have key social relationships been altered or terminated (for example, loss of family member, friend, or staff)?

- Have changes in the person's environment altered access to others or to routine activities (for example, change in apartment, change in room assignment, or change in whom he or she eats with)?

- Have there been changes in the person's access to activity programs (for example, a new problem in locomotion keeps him or her from joining in with others)?

- Have visiting patterns by family, friends, other acquaintances, or volunteers changed?

Treatment and Monitoring

Treatment and monitoring — a multi-aspect approach to care.

- Ensure the person is involved in age-appropriate activities that stimulate and add meaning to life. [See Activities CAP for additional discussion.]

- Treat mood disturbances, psychiatric symptoms, and behavior problems. Focus especially on reducing symptoms of depression.

- If the person has a DRS score of 3 or more, bring him or her to the attention of a physician or mental health professional. This may be an indication of the presence of depression requiring appropriate intervention. [See Mood CAP.]

- Help the person see beyond his or her illness to experience daily life more fully.

- Build upon strengths — extend pleasurable activities, initiate new activities that follow common patterns, increase the presence of those with whom the person feels comfortable.

Facilitate positive social interactions when the person has limited interaction with family and friends.

- Encourage family and friends to be more involved in the person's life.

- Encourage support and care staff to enter into personal exchanges with the person.

- Engage volunteers who are comfortable with the person and who make him or her feel comfortable.

- Find meaningful positive activities for family members and friends to participate in with the person.

- Consult directly with the person to determine what types of social activities he or she likes to engage in as well as those he or she dislikes.

- Encourage others to speak with the person about his or her life. Reminiscing allows the person to reconstruct his or her identity for him- or herself and for others.

Additional Resources

Morris JN, Gwyther L, Gerstein C, Murphy K, Levine D. 1997. Psychosocial well-being. In Morris JN, Lipsitz LA, Murphy KM, and Belleville-Taylor P, eds. *Quality care in the nursing home.* St. Louis, MO: Mosby. **Note:** This chapter provides information on how to conduct an in-depth evaluation of a person's psychosocial well-being as well as strategies for creating opportunities for relationships and activities, interventions to enrich family visits, and approaches to care at the end of life.

Stones MJ, Rattenbury C, Kozma A. 1995. Empirical findings on reminiscence. In Haight BK, Webster J, eds. *The art and science of reminiscing: Theory, research, methods, and applications.* Washington, DC: Taylor & Francis. **Note:** This book provides a scientifically based approach to the use of reminiscence.

Authors

John P. Hirdes, PhD
Michael J. Stones, PhD
Jean-Claude Henrard, MD
John N. Morris, PhD, MSW

Part IV

Clinical Issues CAPs

Falls CAP

Problem

A fall is defined as an unintentional change in position where the person ends up on a lower level (for example, floor, ground, or seat). Falls are a leading cause of morbidity and mortality as persons age and are an important cause of injury among younger vulnerable populations. Interventions that address risk factors for persons who have never fallen focus on multiple goals in areas assumed to be related to falling. These include exercise, balance, delirium, and drug interactions. Multiple CAPs address these issues, but the Falls CAP does not trigger on those who have never fallen. Rather, this CAP focuses on persons who have a higher risk for falling in the future as indicated by a history of prior falls.

Fall rates depend on the frailty of the person, and thus will differ as a function of where the person lives and the service supports received. Over a 6-month period, the expected fall rates differ by residential setting: 40% in long-term care facilities, 35% in home care, and 20 to 30% for older adults living independently in the community. Of those who fall in a 6-month period, most fall only once, and up to 10% of these persons will experience a serious injury — especially hip fractures.

Falls may be an indicator of functional decline and the presence of other conditions, such as delirium, adverse drug reactions, dehydration, and infections. This CAP provides a systematic approach to evaluating a fall, strategies to prevent future falls, and care planning suggestions.

Overall Goals of Care

- Identify and change underlying risk factors for falls.

- Promote activity in a safe manner and in a safe environment.

- Recognize common pathways among falls, incontinence, and functional decline. Fall prevention is not an isolated goal but part of a larger objective of promoting physical activity and improved quality of life.

Falls CAP Trigger

This CAP triggers two groups of persons for specialized follow-up.

TRIGGERED INTO THE HIGH RISK OF FUTURE FALLS GROUP, BASED ON PRIOR REPORT OF A MULTIPLE FALLS

This group includes about 7% of persons in long-term care facilities, 12% of home care recipients, and 3% of older adults living independently in the community. In a long-term care facility setting, about 40% of the persons triggered into this group will fall over a 90-day period. The rate of falls in home care for this same time period tends to be about 65%.

TRIGGERED INTO THE MEDIUM RISK OF FUTURE FALLS GROUP, BASED ON PRIOR REPORT OF A SINGLE FALL

This group includes about 15% of persons in long-term care facilities, 15% of home care recipients, and 10% of older adults living independently in the community. In a long-term care facility setting, about 25% of the persons triggered into this group will fall over a 90-day period. The rate of falls in home care for this same time period tends to be about 40% .

NOT TRIGGERED

No known prior fall. This group includes about 78% of persons in long-term care facilities, 78% of home care recipients, and 83% of older adults living independently in the community.

Falls CAP Guidelines

General Care Plan Considerations

- Have the circumstances of the fall(s) been evaluated?

- Has the person been assessed for the contributing causes of the falls?

- Has the person been assessed for osteoporosis? Is it correctly managed?

- Restraints should be avoided as a fall prevention strategy. They are not associated with a decreased risk of falls or injury associated with falls. The person's right to maintain mobility, despite a slightly elevated risk of falling, should be considered.

- Does the person need a gait, strength, or balance program?

- Has a physician reviewed current medications for their possible effect on falls, including intrinsic contributory factors such as balance, gait, strength, sensory perception, and cognition?

- Is there a program in place to address blood pressure (especially postural changes) and cardiac problems? Has a physician reviewed issues related to blood pressure?

- Has a physician reviewed the possibility of vitamin D deficiency?

Assessment and Care Planning

Common risk factors for falls, other than a history of prior falls, which is by far the best predictor, are outlined in the following list. Each triggered person will likely have one or more of these risk factors. Modifiable risk factors include

- Physical performance limitations: balance, gait, strength, and muscle endurance

- Visual impairment

- Cognitive impairment

- Postural hypotension (with tendency to syncope)

- Cardiac arrhythmia

- Medications (for example, benzodiazepines)

- Environmental factors

- Low levels of physical activity

- Pain from osteoarthritis and other conditions
- Diseases, including Parkinson's disease, epilepsy, diabetes, alcoholism, and stroke
- Vitamin D deficiency

Response to prior fall. A history of falls is the best predictor for future falls. Persons who fall are at a higher risk of falling again, often under similar circumstances. This is particularly true for persons who have had multiple falls. Review the history of falls with the person, family, caregivers, and in the medical/clinical record. Usually a 1-year look-back period is sufficient for this review.

- What were the circumstances of the fall?
  - When did it occur? Night? Day? The exact hour?
  - Did it result in injury?
  - Where did the fall happen? (In the bedroom, bathroom, living room, corridor, on stairs, or outside?)
  - Was it related to taking medications?
- Were any changes to the plan of care made after the fall? Are these changes still applicable to the current situation or does the care plan need updating?

Does the person have limitations in physical performance (balance, gait, muscle strength, and endurance deficits)? Watch for the following indicators of balance problems: sitting, getting up, walking, and turning around. Also, since gait and muscle strength are also related to vitamin D deficiency, this should always be considered.

- Does the person have difficulty maintaining a sitting balance?
- Does the person need to rock his or her body or push off on the arms of a chair when standing up from a chair?
- Does the person have difficulty maintaining a standing position?
- Does the person have a gait problem (for example, unsteady gait even if walking with a mobility aid or personal assistance, slow gait, or takes small steps)?
- Does one leg appear to be shorter than the other, throwing the person off balance when walking?
- Does the person have musculoskeletal problems such as kyphosis (curvature of the spine), weak hip flexors from extended bed rest, or shortening of a leg?
- Does the person have a vitamin D deficiency?

Care Planning Suggestions for Persons Who Need Assistance When Walking or Who Are Nonambulatory

Strategies for improving balance, mobility, and endurance should be incorporated in routine daily activities.

- **Determine if the person can maintain an upright posture for at least 2 minutes without symptoms of light-headedness.** Incorporate into routine activities such as toileting or other daily tasks so that the person is given an opportunity to stand every couple of hours.

(continued)

(continued)

- **For the person who is unsteady, but tries to stand up on his or her own, monitor the person and take the person to the bathroom regularly.** Consider appropriately located grab bars.

- **Walk for exercise a couple of times a day.** Measure distances in the living environment and keep a record of maximum distance walked. Also walk to meals and bathroom as part of the daily routine.

- **Adjust sitting posture in a chair on a regular basis, especially for the person with a tendency to slump down.** When readjusting, offer the person the opportunity to stand and balance, as well as sitting and balancing without leaning on the back of the chair or using armrests for support.

- **Encourage self-propulsion in a wheelchair.** Record the distance the person wheeled by him- or herself or with cueing. (To be successful in wheeling the chair, the wheelchair must be a good fit. Make sure that feet can reach the floor and at least one hand can reach the wheel and the brakes.) The person who can walk with help can increase his or her endurance by wheeling the chair around the living environment using both feet or one leg and one arm.

- **Involve the person in activity programs that provide exercise for balance, muscle strengthening, and flexibility.** Special interventions for physical performance should be considered following a period of low activity due to illness or other change in status, **and** following a fall.

- **Physical activity programs such as those offered at senior centers, YMCAs, community centers, mall walks, tai chi, yoga, and dancing programs are potential activities that may improve or maintain balance.**

Does the person have a visual problem? Visual field deficits, cataracts limiting light perception, and inappropriate eyeglasses are especially common. Review the person's history and assess for the following:

- Has the person been assessed for visual problems, and are there any ophthalmologic diagnoses? Is the care plan up-to-date in terms of medical and environmental treatments for these conditions? Is the person a diabetic?

- Does the person wear eyeglasses for reasons other than reading? Have the eyeglasses been assessed recently to assure satisfactory correction?

- Does the person neglect (appear not to see) objects on one side of the visual field?

- Does poor illumination in the environment affect visual ability?

Care Planning Suggestions for Visual Impairment

- **Ask the person what he or she can see when looking straight ahead.** Know what the person can see in his or her field of vision and place needed objects (for example, mobility aids and dishes) accordingly.

- **Ask the person about his or her ability to differentiate contrasts and surface textures.** Persons with visual impairments may have difficulty detecting changes in levels (for example, stair steps) or the type of surface they are walking on (for example, dry, wet, or icy pavements). Environmental modifications may be useful in some cases (for example, use of tape to mark stair steps). Orientation and mobility training may be offered to support navigation and improve awareness of external environmental conditions.

- **Practice orienting the person to his or her living environment**, keeping in mind what he or she can see. Use visual cueing as reminders and for orientation.

- **Seek advice of occupational therapists for visual cueing.** They have special expertise in treating and providing consultation for neglect of one side of the body or one side of the visual field. These impairments normally result from a stroke.

- **Consider referral to an optometrist or ophthalmologist** if the person has not had an eye examination in the past year.

- **If new visual problems or perceived changes are identified, refer to a physician or optometrist.**

Does the person have a neurological disease, such as Parkinson's disease, with a tremor or rigidity, or a stroke with one-sided weakness?

Does the person have a metabolic disease such as alcoholism or diabetes (hypoglycemia)?

Is the person cognitively impaired (one of the more important risk factors for falls)? Review the person's history and watch for the following:

- Does the person have cognitive performance deficits in memory or everyday decision making?

- Does the person wander? Is the environment safe in which to ambulate?

- Does the person consider him- or herself (or appear to consider him- or herself) able to function at a higher level than he or she is actually capable of? Consider that risky behaviors (standing up alone, getting out of bed alone) are often a result of an unmet need (for example, a need to void). Attending to these needs on a routine basis (for example, by scheduling a toileting plan) may prevent the person from trying risky behaviors. As well, the care provider may need to explore the person's perception and acceptance of his or her physical limitations.

- Review the medications the person is taking. Look for those that can affect the person's level of consciousness, cognitive performance, judgment, and sensory perception.

Care Planning Suggestions for Cognitive Impairment

- **Build wandering about the living environment into exercise-related activities.** Involve the person in purposeful tasks to keep him or her busy and active.

- **Avoid the onset of behaviors** that put the person at risk (for example, address pain, thirst, hunger, and need to toilet).

- **Keep the person active, mobile, and improve balance.** The person with cognitive impairment is less able to learn exercises and learn to use assistive devices for mobility, but he or she can improve with practice and repetition. He or she may take a longer period of time or require greater intensity of intervention to improve. He or she may respond well to activities that he or she did in the past. Find out what activities he or she liked to do.

Medical assessment: Does the person have a problem with blood pressure, an arrhythmia, an especially slow heart beat, or take medictions that may be associated with falls?

- Take heart rate to assess if it is too low or not regular.

- Take blood pressures when the person is lying down, sitting up, and standing to detect orthostatic (postural) hypotension (drop in blood pressure with position changes).

- Compare blood pressures before breakfast and about 20 minutes after breakfast to evaluate for postprandial (after meal) hypotension.

- Is the person taking neuroleptic, anxiolytic, sedative/hypnotic, or antidepressant medications? Does he or she take sleeping pills regularly? If so, for how long has the person been taking these medications? Are medications given regularly or PRN? PRN medications may be associated with a higher risk of falls. If neuroleptics are taken, consider a behavior mapping process to check for side effects.

- Is the person taking cardiovascular medications, COPD medications, or diuretics that might predispose him or her to hypotension?

Care Planning Suggestions for Medical Problems

- **Routinely help/instruct the person to get up from a bed or chair slowly,** allowing for time to balance at the edge of the bed or chair.

- **Consider daily use of support hose.**

- **Encourage the person to avoid large meals** (have more frequent small meals) and/or rest after each meal.

- **Review all medications that can cause blood pressure changes.** Change medication, dose, or timing of dose as indicated. Is the dose timed to minimize negative effects? For example, taking a diuretic in the evening may increase frequency of urination at night; getting out of bed at night places the person at greater risk of falling. Consider a morning dose, if possible.

Review environmental factors that could precipitate a fall.

- Look for hazards and make sure that proper assistive devices and spatial and structural features are in place (for example, grab bars).

Care Planning Suggestions for Environmental Factors

- Assess the environment and provide for

  - Proper lighting for each time of day or night
  - Elimination of glare
  - Proper height of bed and chairs
  - Proper bars, handrails, and devices in bathroom
  - No shine floor/carpet, nonskid strips

- Check hallways, bedrooms, and bathrooms for obstacles.

- People using wheelchairs and walkers need enough space to maneuver safely. A 5-foot (1.5 m) turning radius is considered ideal for most wheelchair users.

- Check for any recent change in the environment (for example, just moved into a new home). If the person has made such a move, has he or she been well oriented to the environment?

- Can the person get into the bathroom with an appropriate mobility aid? (Doorways less than 36 inches [90 cm] wide may be a problem.)

- Should a commode be used at the bedside at night rather than having the person walk to the bathroom in the dark or when half-asleep?

- Is there a need for alternative types of seating — chairs or wheelchairs? Assessment by a therapist can determine the best seating in accordance with the person's physical condition.

- Is the adaptive equipment being used properly?

- Is the assistive device in good condition? Sometimes persons use canes, walkers, and wheelchairs that are not suitable for their size and height. Has the person's status changed, or is there any other reason to believe a new device is needed?

  - Is the device new to the person? Does the person need additional training in how to use the device, when to use it, and what safety procedures must be taken?
  - Are those helping the person aware of how much help or supervision the person needs?

- Check for correct, properly fitted footwear.

If in a long-term care or assisted living facility — after a fall, address immediate health concerns and then review the previously listed risk factors to change and improve the care plan. Observations:

- Compare the vital signs to the person's usual/baseline pattern; be ready to report prior and current vital signs to the physician.

- Prepare an incident report as per facility procedures.

- Contact the physician without delay if any of the following are observed:

  - Abnormal vital signs

  - Suspected dehydration (use BUN/creatinine ratio, if available; otherwise assess for change in urine volume or drinking habits) or infection

  - Change in mental status

  - Change in motor function or speech

  - Inability to resume activity

  - Signs of injury

  - Medications that might have contributed to the fall

  - Alcohol abuse

Care Planning Suggestions after a Fall

- **Consider changes in medications, or timing or dosage of medications.**

- **Consider consults to physical or occupational therapy to assess change in status and plan interventions as needed.**

- **Revise care plan to include additional supervision or a supervised program to help the person resume previous activity levels.** Take into consideration building confidence, modifications in response to potential problems associated with the fall, and any new adaptations due to injuries suffered in the fall.

- If none of the previously listed conditions are present, continue evaluating the circumstances of the fall. Use a consulting pharmacist as a resource in this evaluation, as necessary.

  - Review the person's medications, focusing especially on **new** medication(s), drug dosages, or new combinations of drugs. Review the length of time from the change to the onset of symptoms.

  - Review results of any laboratory tests with the physician.

  - Ask the person to describe how the fall occurred.

  - Evaluate the person for a need to avoid a decline in function secondary to a fall. Injuries, low activity because of illness, or fear of future falls may all contribute to a decline in function. [Review ADL CAP.]

Additional Resources

American Geriatrics Society, British Geriatrics Society, and American Academy of Orthopedic Surgeons. 2001. Panel on fall prevention: Guideline for the prevention of falls in older persons *JAGS* 49: 664–72. **Note:** These comprehensive clinical practice guidelines are the most up-to-date in print and are the results of a collaborative effort between the American Geriatrics Society, the British Geriatrics Society, and the American Association of Orthopedic Surgeons.

American Medical Directors Association. 2003. *Clinical practice guidelines: Falls and fall risk*, 2d ed. Columbia, MD: AMDA.

American Medical Directors Association. 2004. Clinical practice guidelines: Osteoporosis, falls and fall risk. Slide presentation in-service. www.amda.com

Lipsitz LA, Burrows A, Kiel D, Kelley-Gagnon M. 1997. Falls. Morris JN, Lipsitz LA, Murphy KM, Belleville-Taylor P, eds. *Quality care in the nursing home.* St. Louis, MO: Mosby. **Note:** This chapter walks the reader through a step-by-step approach to assessment of persons at risk for falling and provides numerous care planning suggestions.

MacRae PG, Asplund LA, Schnelle JF, Ouslander JG, Abrahase A, Morris C. 1996. A walking program for nursing home persons: Effects on walk endurance, physical activity, mobility, and quality of life. *JAGS* 44: 175–80.

Ray WA, Taylor JA, Meador KG, Thapa PB, Brown AK, Kajihara HK, Davis C, Gideon P, Griffin MR. 1997. A randomized trial of a consultation service to reduce falls in nursing homes. *JAMA* 278: 557–62.

Schnelle JF, MacRae PG, Ouslander JG, Simmons SF, Nitta M. 1995. Functional incidental training, mobility performance, and incontinence care with nursing home persons. *JAGS* 43: 1356–60.

Tinetti ME, Gordon C, Sogolow E, Lapin P, Bradley EH. 2006. Fall-risk evaluation and management: Challenges in adopting geriatric care practices. *The Gerontologist* 46: 717–25.

Authors

Katherine Berg, PhD, PT
Lewis A. Lipsitz, MD
Palmi V. Jonsson, MD
Margaret Kelley-Gagnon, RN
Beryl D. Goldman, PhD, RN
Katharine M. Murphy, PhD, RN
John N. Morris, PhD, MSW
Katarzyna Szczerbińska, MD, PhD
Knight Steel, MD

Pain CAP

Problem

Pain is defined as "an unpleasant sensory and emotional experience associated with actual or potential tissue damage." It is a subjective experience, and "the inability to communicate verbally does not negate the possibility that an individual is experiencing pain and is in need of appropriate pain-relieving treatment" (International Association for the Study of Pain — IASP).

Pain can be affected by damage to various physiologic systems and tissues, including musculoskeletal (for example, arthritis, fractures, injury from peripheral vascular disease, wounds), neurological (for example, diabetic neuropathy, herpes zoster), and cancer. The intensity (severity) of the pain is a subjective matter and is not necessarily proportional to the type or extent of tissue or system damage.

Among the relevant issues assessed in the Pain CAP are the newness of the pain, the intensity of the pain, the nature of current treatments, and the extent to which self-reported pain is hindered by cognitive or communication deficits.

The presence of pain can also increase suffering in other areas, leading to an increased sense of helplessness, anxiety, depression, decreased activity, decreased appetite, and disrupted sleep. Management of pain thus extends beyond analgesia to include other interventions and treatments focusing on the person's quality of life and ability to function.

Pain must be managed in a timely fashion, especially if it is of recent onset. Pain management should involve an interdisciplinary approach, working with the person and his or her family or caregiver. Additionally, to be effective, the informal caregivers and the person must communicate the signs and symptoms of pain in a timely manner to the physician and other members of the care team.

Overall Goals of Care

- Identify and treat underlying reasons for pain.
- Optimize the ability to perform activities of daily living and to live an active social life.
- Relieve suffering.
- Monitor treatment efficacy and adverse effects.
- Recognize the association of pain and other issues, such as depression, withdrawal, and functional decline. Pain management should be viewed as part of a larger objective promoting physical activity and quality of life.

17

Pain CAP Trigger

This CAP applies to long-term care, home care, assisted living, post-acute care, and community health assessment. The goal of this CAP is to assess and manage pain and the problems it causes in a timely fashion.

This CAP triggers two groups of persons for specialized follow-up, based on the severity of the reported pain rather than the likelihood of curing the pain. In fact, it is relatively uncommon that a person in either triggered group will be fully cured. Thus, the key goal of this CAP is to improve the person's general status.

HIGH RISK TRIGGER

A person with severe, horrible, or excruciating pain (whether the pain occurs daily or less frequently). This group includes about 5% of persons in long-term care facilities, 25% of home care recipients, and 4% of older adults living independently in the community. In a long-term care facility setting, about 45% of the persons triggered into this group will improve over a 90-day period, and 15% will become pain free. The rate of improvement in home care is about 15%, while the proportion becoming pain free is only about 5%.

MEDIUM RISK TRIGGER

A person with daily pain described as mild or moderate. This group includes about 12% of persons in long-term care facilities, 25% of home care recipients, and 15% of older adults living independently in the community. In a long-term care facility setting, about 35% of the persons triggered into this group will improve over a 90-day period, and 15% will become pain free. The rate of improvement in home care is about 14%, while the proportion becoming pain free again is about 7%.

NOT TRIGGERED

All other persons.

Pain CAP Guidelines

Further Assessment of Pain

Pain frequency and intensity. To manage pain, a thorough assessment includes the following:

1. taking a detailed history of pain intensity, location, frequency, and characteristics;

2. completing an accurate physical examination;

3. carrying out proper laboratory studies;

4. deciding the extent to which the pain affects emotional status and preferences;

5. observing the performance of the person; and

6. reviewing present interventions and assessing their efficacy and side effects, if any.

Additional considerations in assessing pain:

■ Do not assume that changes in pain patterns or new pain are caused by pre-existing conditions. A new, thorough evaluation should be carried out each time there is new pain or a change in the pattern of existing pain.

■ As pain is common in older adults and persons living with chronic illness, pain should be treated as the fifth vital sign and, as such, monitored on a regular and scheduled basis.

■ After the assessment with an interRAI instrument, follow up by asking the person to grade the pain severity using a supplemental pain assessment tool the person finds easy to use (examples are provided in the text that follows). Include the person's estimate of pain intensity at its lowest and highest levels. Questions should be simple and concrete, and the person's statements about pain should be taken at face value. If the person does not understand, use simpler or different words. Use the interRAI pain questions regularly, as well as any supplemental tools, to check pain symptoms over time. Record findings on a pain flow sheet to assess the efficacy of interventions. Examples of supplemental pain assessment tools include the visual analog scale (person places a mark on a 10 cm line in accordance to severity); a numerical rating scale (how bad the pain is on a scale of 0, no pain, to 10, worst possible pain); the verbal descriptive scale (mild, moderate, severe, horrible, excruciating); and the faces pain scale (showing faces from a smiling one to a face in extreme agony). There are also specialized pain assessment tools for persons with difficulties in verbalization.

- For persons on an analgesic, a routine pain reassessment is recommended. This will help you titrate the analgesic as necessary.

Observe frequency and intensity of pain. To manage pain adequately, continuing observation of the person's performance is important. If the person cannot communicate verbally, lacks the ability to describe symptoms, or tends not to complain, observation is the only way to assess pain.

You should be sensitive to cultural factors that may affect the manifestation of pain. For some cultural groups, a tendency toward stoicism may hinder the person's willingness to express pain. On the other hand, there may be a tendency for staff or informal caregivers to inappropriately discount pain indicators among persons who are more expressive about health concerns than expected based on cultural norms.

Use observations during usual activities (for example, morning care, physical therapy) to establish or confirm the person's pain complaints/signs of pain, and correlate this with changes in physical functioning. Speak with those providing direct care, including family members, and document the observations of these individuals.

Nonverbal signs of pain:

- facial expressions (for example, frowning, grimacing)

- vocal behaviors (for example, sighing, moaning)

- body position (for example, guarding, distorted posture, restricted limb movement, increased resting)

- change in routine (for example, staying in bed, less or slowed involvement in activities of daily living, decreased intake of food and fluids)

- change in mental status (for example, irritability, confusion)

- signs of aggression

Determine pain location, type, and response to external conditions. Determine as precisely as possible where the person feels pain. Where the pain is located can be of importance when the care plan is developed (for example, pain related to peripheral vascular disease or arthritis will affect the care planning interventions).

- Find out if the pain is constant, changes over time, or comes and goes (intermittent). If intermittent, ask about its frequency, duration, and the circumstances in which it occurrs. The person's pain experience may vary by site, time of day, and activity.

- Ask the person to describe what the pain feels like. Ask: "What words best describe it?" Descriptions may be helpful in guiding therapy and in finding out whether the pain is more likely neuropathic (burning, pins and needles, shooting, numbness), musculoskeletal (cramping, crushing, throbbing, stabbing), or visceral (cramping, tightness).

- Ask what makes the pain better or worse (for example, moving, sitting still, staying in the same position, following medication administration, maintaining drug schedule, taking medication as pain arises). Has the pain subsided as hoped following the implementation of a planned analgesic drug program? Note what behavior seems to relieve the pain and what makes it worse.

All information from this discussion must be correlated to findings from the physical examination and proper laboratory data.

Assess treatment preferences. Discuss treatment choices with the person (and family as appropriate) and ask about preferences and expectations. Respecting preferences promotes adherence to a regimen and achievement of therapeutic goals. For example, it is not uncommon for terminally ill persons, preparing for end of life, to prefer experiencing some pain rather than taking doses of medication that result in a diminished level of alertness.

Management of Pain

Pharmacological Intervention

Consider whether the person prefers to be (or should be) referred to a pain clinic or pain outreach team. The treating physician usually prescribes a drug therapy after identifying new pain or an acute flare-up of chronic pain. A person may be in daily pain for long periods without a drug regimen being prescribed, but this must not be permitted to occur. Before starting a new medication, identify and review all medications the person is taking, including over-the-counter medications, alternative medications, and herbal remedies. It is also important to set a specific pain improvement goal, responding to the person's desired comfort level within a specified time period.

The physician does not always have the same opportunity as other clinical staff (for example, nurses) or family members to monitor the results of the intervention on the person's everyday life. Therefore, the nurses and family members are in a key position to interview the person and observe the impact of new medications. The person and the nearest caregivers should be aware of what pain medication has been started and the strength of its effect (where it stands on the analgesic ladder introduced by the World Health Organization [WHO]; (see box on next page), how soon the medication can be expected to show its effect, and what adverse effects to monitor. [See Appropriate Medications CAP.]

Drug therapy is a mainstay for managing pain. Adhere to these basic concepts of treatment:

- By mouth is the most convenient and cost-effective route of administration.

- By the clock involves around-the-clock administration, rather than as needed, and allows each analgesic dose to achieve constant pain control. However, for control of severe pain, self-administered pain medication (for example, a patient-controlled morphine pump) often results in more acceptable levels of pain control with lower use of the analgesic.

- By the ladder administration is modified from the WHO Three-Step Analgesic Ladder (see box on next page). Note that in addition to traditional analgesic medications, several other types of pharmaceuticals have pain-relieving effects. Consider consulting the physician about how to improve pain management by elevating the pain threshold (that is, the point at which a person is uncomfortable with his or her pain) with the use of antidepressants or managing neuropathic pain.

■ Choose the best single analgesic for the person, then titrate the dose up or down as necessary. Side effects are easier to identify if only one drug is initially provided. At the same time, choosing the single best analgesic may be quite difficult. Many pharmaceutical agents are now being co-formulated to better control pain (the key for breakthrough pain is to prescribe very rapidly available substances).

■ Increase the drug dose or strength (in the case of opioids) when there is inadequate pain control. Often, an additional one-third of the present dose of opioid is added to control breakthrough pain.

■ Prevent and treat analgesic side effects. Precautions must be taken with some medications to control unwanted side effects (WHO Ladder — see box). Side effects are more likely to occur in older and frailer persons with adverse effects often arising from changes in the central nervous system (for example, delirium, restlessness, sleepiness). Other common symptoms are gastrointestinal (for example, nausea, vomiting, stomach irritation, constipation).

Adapted from the WHO LADDER for Chronic Pain

For mild to moderate pain:
Step 1: "nonopioids": Paracetamol/Acetaminophen, aspirin, or other nonsteroidal anti-inflammatory drugs (NSAIDs — **Note:** While this is in the WHO approach, many geriatric pain experts might take NSAIDs off this list considering their potential for side effects, including GI, renal, delirium); start ulcer prophylaxis.

If moderate pain remains unrelieved by Step 1 drugs:
Step 2: "weak" opioids; start laxatives (unless contraindicated).

For moderate to severe pain unrelieved by Step 2 drugs:
Step 3: "strong" opioids; start laxatives (unless contraindicated), consider medications for nausea, if needed. **Note:** The distinction between weak and strong opioids, although still widely used, is not state of the art. Strong opioids at Step 3 are now commonly classified as Step 2 level agents, exactly as the "weak" opioids, because they are co-formulated at very low dosages with other agents.

Nonpharmacological Intervention

Nonpharmacological approaches are important in pain management because they

■ may augment the efficacy of medications

■ usually have minimal adverse effects

■ give the person and family a sense of participation and control

■ may address functional decline, mood, and social isolation

Educate the person, family, and direct care staff.

■ Dispel myths that pain and disability are normal parts of aging.

■ Discuss the cause of the pain, pain assessment findings, goals of treatment, multidisciplinary plan of care, prognosis, treatment options, and side effects.

Consider the following approaches:

- Physical, occupational, and other therapies to help with safety assessment (for example, falls, injuries), immobilization of a joint, strength and endurance training, and other pain management techniques.

- Physical modalities (for example, heat, ice, or massage).

- Relaxation and distraction techniques (for example, individual, group, or one-on-one activities, such as meditation, music, conversation, or audio books).

- Other options include acupuncture, tai chi, and other complementary therapies.

- Help the person set realistic and concrete goals (for example, walk 100 feet, go to an activity three times a week).

- Consider whether the person needs added psychological and social support.

Prevention of Unwanted Consequences of Pain

- Special attention should be paid to the relationship between pain and functional capacity. [See ADL CAP.]

- Special attention should be given to the relationship between pain and depression. Persons in chronic pain tend to develop depression, and therefore they should always be assessed for depression. [See Mood CAP, specifically Depression Rating Scale, and remember that the relationship between pain and depression is bi-directional.]

- Active management of underlying and accompanying diseases.

- To prevent other negative consequences of pain, see Behavior CAP and Social Relationship CAP.

Additional Resources

American Geriatric Society Panel on Chronic Pain in Older Persons. 1998. The management of chronic pain in older persons. *JAGS* 46(5): 635–51.

Bair MJ, Robinson RL, Katon W, Kroenke K. 2003. Depression and pain comorbidity. *Arch Intern Med* 163: 2433–45.

Bernabei R, Gambassi G, Lapane K, et al. 1998. Management of pain in elderly persons with cancer. *JAMA* 279(23): 1877–82. **Note:** This paper describes the prevalence and predictors of daily cancer pain and analgesic treatment using MDS pain and drug data from five states. Findings: 26% of persons in pain received no treatment; others were inadequately treated, especially older and minority persons.

Farrell MJ, Katz B, Helme RD. 1996. The impact of dementia on the pain experience. *Pain* 67: 7–15.

Finne-Soveri UH, Ljunggren G, Schroll M, Jonsson PV, Hjaltadottir I, El Kholy K, Tilvis RS. 2000. Pain and its association with disability in the institutional long-term care in four Nordic countries. *The Canadian Journal on Aging* (Suppl 2) 19: S38–49.

Scherder E, Oosterman J, Swaab D, Herr K, Ooms M, Ribbe M, Sergeant J, Pickering G, Benedetti F. 2005. Recent developments in pain in dementia. *BMJ* 330: 461–64.

Stolee P, Hillier LM, Esbaugh J, Bol McKellar L, Gauthier N. 2005. Instruments for the assessment of pain in older persons with cognitive impairment. *JAGS* 53: 319–26.

Zyxzkowsa J, Szczerbińska K, Jantzi MR, Hirdes JP. 2007. Pain among the oldest old in community and institutions. *Pain* 129(1-2): 167–76. Epub 2007, January 23.

Clinical Practice Guidelines, Manuals, and Web Sites

American Pain Society. A multidisciplinary educational and scientific organization serving people in pain by advancing research, education, treatment, and professional practice. www.ampainsoc.org

City of Hope Pain Resource Center. Serves as a clearinghouse to disseminate resources to help institutions improve pain management. Over 300 materials can be found on this site. http://prc.coh.org

Griffie J, Matson S, Muchka S, Weissman D. 1998. Improving pain in the long-term care setting: A resource guide for institutional change. Medical College of Wisconsin, Milwaukee, WI. Division of Hematology/Oncology, 9200 W. Wisconsin Ave., Milwaukee, WI 53226. (414) 805-4605.

Griffie J, Muchka S, Weissman D. 2000. Nursing staff education resource manual: Pain management 101: A six session in-service education program in pain management for long-term care facilities. Medical College of Wisconsin, Milwaukee, WI. Division of Hematology/Oncology, 9200 W. Wisconsin Ave., Milwaukee, WI 53226. (414) 805-4605.

International Association for the Study of Pain: www.iasp-pain.org

McCaffery M, Pasero C. 1999. *Pain: Clinical manual.* St. Louis, MO: C.V. Mosby.

Palliative Medicine Program at the Medical College of Wisconsin. Develops, implements, and disseminates innovative educational and clinical care programs. This Web site offers resource materials, analgesic guidelines, and information on institutional pain management. www.mcw.edu/pallmed

Rochon T, Patry G, DeSilva D. 2001. *Pain relief resource manual.* Brown University Center for Gerontology and Health Care Research, Providence, RI. (401) 863-9628.

U.S. Department of Health and Human Services. 1992. *Clinical practice guidelines: Acute pain management.* (AHCPR Publication No. 92-0032). Washington, DC: U.S. Government Printing Office. (Also available online at www.nlm.nih.gov)

U.S. Department of Health and Human Services. 1994. *Clinical practice guidelines: Management of cancer pain.* (AHCPR Publication No. 94-0592). Washington, DC: U.S. Government Printing Office. (Also available online at www.nlm.nih.gov)

Authors

Aida Won, MD
Harriet Finne-Soveri, MD, PhD
Dinnus Frijters, PhD
Giovanni Gambassi, MD
Katharine M. Murphy, PhD, RN
John N. Morris, PhD, MSW

Pressure Ulcer CAP

Problem

A pressure ulcer is defined as a localized injury to the skin and/or underlying tissue usually over a bony prominence, as a result of pressure, or pressure in combination with shear and/or friction (from www.npuap.org). A number of contributing or confounding factors are also associated with pressure ulcers; the significance of these factors is yet to be elucidated.

Pressure ulcers occur because of pressure over a localized area of skin. They can be limited to the skin or they may involve deep tissues including the underlying bone. They are graded (or described) according to depth. Often they are found over a bony prominence, especially the sacrum and the greater trochanter (upper part of the femur).

If a pressure ulcer is not present, the goal is to prevent one from occurring. If a pressure ulcer is present, the goal is to heal or close it. Unfortunately, these goals cannot always be accomplished. Nevertheless, every effort should be made to do so.

The higher the pressure ulcer descriptive stage, the more severe and the longer the recovery period is likely to be. Healing may be protracted, labor-intensive, and expensive. The following staging (or grading) system is used widely to describe the severity of skin breakdown.

- Stage 1: An observable pressure-related change of intact skin that may include changes in one or more of the following: skin temperature (warmth or coolness), tissue consistency (firm or boggy feel), or sensation (pain, itching). The ulcer appears as a defined area of persistent redness in lightly pigmented skin, whereas in darker skins, the ulcer may appear with persistent red, blue, or purple hues, or its color may simply differ from the surrounding area.

- Stage 2: Partial skin loss involving epidermis, dermis, or both. The ulcer is superficial and presents clinically as an abrasion, open blister, or shallow crater.

- Stage 3: Full thickness skin loss involving damage or necrosis (death of cells) of subcutaneous tissue that may extend down to, but not through, underlying fascia. Bone, tendon, or muscle are not exposed. The ulcer presents clinically as a deep crater with or without undermining of adjacent tissue.

- Stage 4: Full thickness skin loss with extensive tissue necrosis or damage to muscle, bone, or supporting structures (for example, tendon, joint capsule). Undermining and sinus tracts also may be associated with stage 4 ulcers.

- Stage undetermined (for new suite of interRAI tools only): Unstageable often as ulcer is covered with necrotic tissue.

Some of the negative outcomes of pressure ulcers are pain and suffering, increased risk for infections or infecting others, and mortality. A person with a pressure ulcer has three times the mortality risk of a person without an ulcer.

Overall Goals of Care

- Prevent pressure ulcers from occurring.

- Optimize the local wound or skin environment, allowing the ulcer to close.

- Achieve a clean ulcer base with granulation tissue.

- Maintain a moist local skin environment to allow granulation to take place.

- Check the progress of pressure ulcer healing.

- Prevent the development of more severe or new pressure ulcers.

- Check skin regularly for signs of emerging pressure ulcers.

Pressure Ulcer CAP Trigger

This CAP trigger identifies three subgroups of persons for specialized follow-up. The specialized follow-up seeks to heal either an existing pressure ulcer or to prevent pressure ulcers from occurring. Specialized follow-up may include consultation with a practitioner (physician, wound care specialist, or nurse) with expertise in ulcer/wound care.

TRIGGERED — HAS A STAGE 2 OR HIGHER LEVEL PRESSURE ULCER AND THE GOAL OF CARE IS HEALING

The proportion of persons with such a pressure ulcer in any service program in part depends on the vigilance of the caregivers (staff) in preventing pressure ulcers.

In long-term care facilities the range can be wide, with some facilities having few persons with a stage 2 or higher pressure ulcer, and others having many persons with this condition. On average, about 10% of persons in long-term care facilities fall into this category, including those who entered the facility with an ulcer.

In a home care program, 2 to 8% of persons will have a stage 2 or higher stage pressure ulcer. Among older adults living independently in the community, this condition is uncommon.

Care outcomes. Over a 90-day period, about 60% of persons in long-term care facilities with a stage 2 or higher pressure ulcer will improve, while about 45% of home care recipients will improve.

TRIGGERED — DOES NOT HAVE A STAGE 2 OR HIGHER PRESSURE ULCER BUT IS AT RISK OF DEVELOPING SUCH AN ULCER

Two subgroups of persons fall into this category.

TRIGGERED — HAS A STAGE 1 PRESSURE ULCER

Over a 90-day period, the proportion of persons who will progress to a stage 2, or higher, pressure ulcer varies by the type of program the person is in. About 4% of persons in long-term care facilities and about the same percentage of home care recipients fall into this group. Less commonly, older adults living independently in the community fall into this group.

Care outcomes. In long-term care facilities, about 15% of those triggered into this group will progress to having a stage 2 or higher pressure ulcer over the next 90 days; in a home care program, about 7% will so decline. At the same time, many more of those with a stage 1 pressure ulcer will have no pressure ulcer 90 days later — about 67% of persons in long-term care facilities and 45% of home care recipients.

Dependent, or activity did not occur in either bed mobility or transfer, **and** has one or more of the following risk factors present: has a history of pressure ulcers, has an indwelling catheter, has a stasis ulcer, or is receiving wound care. About 4% of persons in long-term care facilities, 3% of home care recipients, and less than 1% of older adults living independently in the community fall into this risk group.

Care outcomes. About 15% of persons in long-term care facilities and 10% of home care recipients with the above risk factors will develop a pressure ulcer over the following 90-day period.

NOT TRIGGERED

Has no pressure ulcer or pressure ulcer risk factors. This subgroup includes 82% of persons in long-term care facilities, 90% of home care recipients, and 99% of older adults living independently in the community.

Pressure Ulcer CAP Guidelines

Ulcer Management

For all ulcers present at admission into a program, document the following: location, size, stage, presence and type of drainage, presence of odors, and description of the surrounding skin. If possible, take a picture of the ulcer.

Is an eschar (blackened devitalized tissue) present? Is yellow tissue (slough) present?

- A physician or wound care specialist consultation is needed to determine how (and by whom and where) to remove this tissue or if it should be removed. Debridement choices to remove the damaged and dead tissue include surgical and chemical means.

Does the wound bed seem infected?

- If there is reason to believe the ulcer is infected (such as the presence of a foul odor, increasing pain, surrounding skin is reddened [erythema] or warm, or there is a presence of pus) treatment options to be considered by the physician or wound care specialist include

  - Topical or systemic antibiotics

  - Debridement

  - In chronic wounds, silver impregnated dressings may be a better choice given the increased incidence of antibiotic resistant organisms.

Is granulation tissue present (a beefy red tissue resulting from new capillary formation and fibroblasts)? This is essential for healing to occur.

- View the wound at the time any wound care product is applied and note whether granulation tissue is present and the wound is healing as expected.

  - If the condition of the wound bed begins to decline, a physician or wound care expert consultation is needed.

- Once granulation tissue is present, the goal is to maintain a clean, moist environment. Some products that may be helpful include

  - Polymer films and foams

  - Hydrogels

  - Hydrocolloids

- Alginates or absorptive beads
- Combination products
- Silver impregnated products

- Document the depth of the ulcer and measure it at least weekly. Record the presence of granulation tissue, slough, eschar, or signs of an infection. Employ a progress monitoring tool.

If the ulcer does not show signs of healing, despite therapy, consider complicating factors.

- Is there an elevated bacterial level in the absence of clinical infection? Is exudate present, necrotic debris or slough in the wound, too much granulation tissue, or odor in the wound bed? Expert consultation should be considered if these conditions are present.

- Is there an underlying osteomyelitis (bone infection)? Additional diagnostic studies may be needed.

- Are there co-morbid conditions or illnesses? Many acute and chronic conditions, such as diabetes mellitus, a malignancy, or the use of steroids, may make healing difficult.

- Is the person terminally ill? Consider changing treatment goals to comfort measures.

- Has a turning schedule been implemented? This should remove pressure from the wound but should also minimize pressure on areas at risk.

- Does the person need a pressure relieving or reducing mattress? Consultation may be needed for the appropriate surface.

- Have nutritional deficits been addressed? Although data on the efficacy are limited, consider vitamins and minerals (for example, zinc and vitamin C) supplementation. [See Undernutrition CAP.]

- Is protein intake sufficient for healing? Generally about 1.25 grams of protein per kg of body weight is recommended if there are no contraindications to this diet. Has a dietitian been consulted? [See Undernutrition CAP.]

- Is pain present when dressings are changed? Evaluate for underlying infection and bone or tissue involvement. [See Pain CAP.]

- Is the person depressed or frustrated by the ulcer? Consider counseling, if appropriate, to the person and/or family/caregivers regarding the treatment plan and its potentially protracted course. [See Mood CAP.]

For those at risk of developing pressure ulcers, treat as follows:

Evaluate for extrinsic risk factors.

- Pressure
  - Can the person move sufficiently to relieve pressure over any one site? If not, must a caregiver move the person?
  - Is the person confined to a bed or chair all or most of the time?
  - Is the mattress or seat cushion appropriate to reduce or relieve pressure? Can a special pressure relieving mattress or chair cushion be provided?
  - If the person cannot move independently, is a regular (for example, every 2 hours) turning schedule provided?

- Ensure that the person and family understand the need to monitor pressure points.

- Friction and shearing forces

  - Is the person sliding down in the bed?

  - Is the person who needs help with bed mobility or transfer moved by sliding rather than lifting?

- Maceration (destruction of skin because of excess moisture)

  - Is the person persistently wet, especially from fecal incontinence, wound drainage, or perspiration?

Evaluate for intrinsic risk factors.

- Altered mental status

  - Is delirium limiting mobility? [See Delirium CAP.]

  - Is cognitive loss limiting mobility? [See Cognitive Loss CAP.]

  - Address the underlying cause(s) of mental status changes to the extent possible.

- Immobility (person is unable to change position)

  - Is it because of a condition such as a stroke, multiple sclerosis, or hip fracture?

  - Has physical or occupational therapy been maximized?

  - Is immobility due to other causes?

    - Physical restraints should always be removed unless the person is at serious risk of self-injury or injury to others and no other means of control is possible. [See Physical Restraints CAP.]
    - Consider reducing the dose of or stopping medications that limit mobility (for example, psychotropics, opioids). Review all medications with the physician (or the nurse-practitioner or physician assistant) and consulting pharmacist. [See Medication CAP.]

- Incontinence: Fecal incontinence may be associated with pressure ulcer formation. [See Bowel CAP.]

  - Has a scheduled toileting program been tried?

- Poor nutrition [See Undernutrition CAP.]

- Have additional disease states, for example, peripheral vascular disease, diabetes mellitus, and any cause of decreased sensation been discussed with the physician or appropriate health care provider?

- Inactivity

  - What is limiting the person's degree of physical activity?

Additional Resources

Baranoski S, Ayello EA. 2003. *Wound care essentials: Practice principals.* Springhouse, PA: Springhouse. **Note:** A practical guide to wound care, especially pressure ulcers.

Bergstrom N, Bennett MA, Carlson CE, et al. 1994. Treatment of pressure ulcers. *Clinical practice guideline*, no. 15. Rockville, MD: U.S. Department of Health and Human Services. Public Health Service, Agency for Health Care

Policy and Research. AHCPR Publication No. 95-0652. **Note:** Extensive literature review and grading of the evidence regarding treatment.

Brandeis GH, Powell JW. 1997. Pressure ulcers. In Morris JN, Lipsitz LA, Murphy KM, Belleville-Taylor P, eds. *Quality care in the nursing home.* St. Louis, MO: Mosby, 303–14. **Note:** This chapter provides an overview of pressure ulcers with emphasis for the nursing home person.

European Pressure Ulcer Advisory Panel (EPUAP): www.epuap.org

Folkedahl BA, Frantz RA, Goode C. 2002. *Treatment of pressure ulcers: Research-based protocol.* The University of Iowa, Gerontological Nursing Interventions Research, Research Dissemination Care. **Note:** This protocol provides helpful information for assessing and monitoring pressure ulcers and risk factors for development. www.nursing.uiowa.edu

Hess CT. 2004. *Clinical guide: Wound care.* Philadelphia, PA: Lippincott, Williams and Wilkins. **Note:** A practical guide to wound care, especially pressure ulcers.

National Pressure Ulcer Advisory Panel. Pressure Ulcer Scale for Healing (PUSH) Tool version 3.0. 9/15/98. **Note:** The PUSH tool is copyright by NUPAP. www.npuap.org

National Pressure Ulcer Advisory Panel. Supplementary Surface Standards, Terms and Definitions 8/29/2006. Internet address: www.npuap.org

Reddy, R, Sudeeo, SG, Rochon, PA. 2006. Preventing pressure ulcers: A systematic review. *JAMA* 296:974–84.

Registered Nurses Association of Ontario (RNAO). 2002. Assessment and management of stage I to IV pressure ulcers. (August) 104 pp. [70 references].

Thomas DR. 1997. Pressure ulcers. In Cassel CK, Cohen HJ, Larson EB, et al., eds. *Geriatric medicine,* 3d ed. New York: Springer. 767–84. **Note:** General review of the subject of pressure ulcers.

Authors

Gary H. Brandeis, MD
Harriet Finne-Soveri, MD, PhD
John N. Morris, PhD, MSW
Sue Nonemaker, RN, MS
Knight Steel, MD
Pauline Belleville-Taylor, RN, MS, CS

Cardiorespiratory Conditions CAP

Problem

The Cardiorespiratory Conditions CAP alerts the health care professional to the need to assess and manage the person for possible cardiovascular or respiratory problems. Many, but not all, adults who have cardiorespiratory difficulties will already be under the care of a physician. In addition, some persons may develop new symptoms or an exacerbation of old symptoms that require medical or other intervention.

The prevalence of heart disease increases rapidly with age. In Western societies, 75% of all persons with heart failure are 60 years of age or older, and 20% or more of persons 75 years of age or older have a history of a heart attack or angina. Many older persons with hypertension may develop symptoms from an abrupt change in blood pressure or a new medication. Chronic obstructive pulmonary disease (COPD) is widespread especially in those who have smoked or who have worked in certain industries.

Some signs and symptoms, such as shortness of breath or chest pain associated with exertion, may be clearly attributable to the cardiorespiratory systems. However, in some cases such as general fatigue, the relationship to the cardiorespiratory systems may not be immediately apparent. Furthermore, signs and symptoms of acute illness, such as pneumonia, may be difficult to recognize in the presence of a chronic condition such as COPD. All such problems can severely restrict a person's lifestyle and should be monitored and addressed.

Overall Goals of Care

- Help nonphysicians working with older adults in the community identify potential cardiovascular or respiratory symptoms.
- Refer to a physician and other health professionals those who exhibit signs and symptoms of cardiovascular or respiratory difficulties and are not already under active care.

Cardiorespiratory Conditions CAP Triggers

Cardiovascular and respiratory disease in older adults may or may not be under treatment and the person may or may not have participated in cardiopulmonary self-management or other intervention programs. Limitation in functioning may not be recognized as being due to cardiorespiratory disease or may be attributed to the onset of old age. Many symptoms, such as shortness of breath, may be accepted and tolerated. Thus, this CAP identifies whether the symptom is present without first excluding those who may already be under a physician's care.

TRIGGERED   Persons who display any of the following symptoms:

- Chest pain
- Shortness of breath

- Irregular pulse

- Dizziness

- Presence of any of the following test results. (These items do not appear on the interRAI assessment forms and are available only if you or the physician ordered or completed the test. Also, they should not be taken as normal limits.)

  - Systolic blood pressure > 200 or < 100 mmHG

  - Respiratory rate > 20 per minute

  - Heart rate > 100 or < 50 per minute

  - Oxygen saturation < 94%

This triggered group includes 15% of persons in long-term care facilities, about 40% of persons receiving home care (9% with chest pain, 25% with shortness of breath, 15% with irregular pulse, and 20% with dizziness), and 35% of older adults living independently in the community (4% with chest pain, 15% with shortness of breath, 10% with irregular pulse, and 20% with dizziness).

NOT TRIGGERED   Persons who do not have any of the previously mentioned symptoms.

Cardiorespiratory Conditions CAP Guidelines

It is important to ensure that cardiorespiratory symptoms are evaluated. Many persons with such symptoms will require urgent attention, and there are many therapeutic options to treat these conditions, depending on the cause of the symptoms. Heart failure, for example, usually responds to treatment for a considerable period of time, leading to an improved quality of life in terms of exercise tolerance and degree of fatigue. In addition, some symptoms may not be immediately recognized as resulting from cardiovascular disease. For example, light-headedness, dizziness, or blackouts (syncope), often related to a drop in blood pressure, may also be the result of abnormalities of a heart valve or an arrhythmia, both of which may be amenable to medical or surgical intervention.

Frequently, persons may have both cardiovascular and respiratory illnesses. The principal symptoms and signs associated with cardiovascular and respiratory disease are as follows:

- **Cardiovascular disease** — Shortness of breath (dyspnea), chest pain, palpitations, swelling of the lower extremities, light-headedness, dizziness, blackouts (syncope).

- **Respiratory disease** — Shortness of breath, cough, sputum production, coughing up blood, wheezing, and chest pain. Sometimes persons simply say that "they cannot get enough air." To determine the cause of one of these symptoms or signs, a thorough medical examination is required.

When present, ask the person whether a physician is aware of the problem and whether the person is under treatment for the condition. Regardless of the answer, suggest that the presence of these symptoms warrants further discussion with the physician.

The following material provides further information on these symptoms. It is provided to assist the clinician in discussing the problem with the person. But remember, the principal goal is to convince the person to see a physician.

Irregular pulse. A new irregular pulse always requires evaluation. If, for example, it is a reflection of atrial fibrillation, the person has an increased risk of stroke. However, this is just one of many causes of an irregular pulse.

Cough, sputum production, and wheezing. Cough, with or without sputum production, is initiated when the lining of the respiratory tract is irritated and is by far the most common respiratory symptom. Cough is commonly caused by upper respiratory infections of a viral nature. Sputum associated with infection, especially of a bacterial nature, often is colored and thick and viscous. Brown, pink, or dark coloration may be due to blood. Bloody sputum may result from an acute infection, a chronic one (for example, tuberculosis), a tumor, blood clots in the lungs, and a lengthy list of other conditions that always require medical evaluation. In addition, cough may be caused by a medication, most commonly one recommended for the treatment of hypertension or congestive heart failure. Nearly all heavy smokers have a chronic cough. Other causes include pneumonia, bronchitis, congestive heart failure (CHF), mild asthma, and, rarely, tumors. People with asthma or chronic lung disease, such as emphysema, may also complain of wheezing, which is a sense of difficulty moving air, especially on breathing out, often associated with an audible sound. If new in onset or severe, it requires urgent medical attention.

Similarly an increase in sputum production or a change in the character of the sputum needs to be evaluated by a physician.

Chest pain. Chest pain always requires a thorough medical evaluation. The cause often, but not always, may be able to be determined by a detailed history and physical examination. Usually, however, one or more blood tests and perhaps a radiologic study or even an endoscopic study as well as an electrocardiogram are needed to confirm the diagnosis.

The typical pain of heart (ischemic) disease is a squeezing, gripping pain. It is often felt in the center of the chest, but may be noted in the throat, one or both arms, the jaw and lower teeth, or even the back. The pain may be associated with exertion or palpitations and may reoccur under similar circumstances. When mild it may barely be noticed or incorrectly attributed to indigestion. It may persist or it may be transient. There are many other causes of chest pain that may be confused with pain originating in the heart, including esophageal disease, a chest infection, a pulmonary embolism (blood clot lodging in the lung), dissection of the aorta (tearing of the wall of this artery), and arthritis in the neck or back. Chest pain therefore requires an immediate medical evaluation. It is of particular concern when new in onset or when becoming worse, increasing in frequency, occurring at rest, of prolonged duration (longer than 10 minutes), or when it is associated with other symptoms or signs such as light-headedness or difficulty breathing.

Syncope or blackout. Sudden collapse with loss of consciousness and spontaneous recovery (fainting or syncope) often is caused by a cardiovascular problem, such as a heart attack or an arrhythmia. Other common causes include a drop in blood pressure (hypotension) associated with blood loss, dehydration, a postural change, medications or a change in a medication, a cardiovascular reflex after coughing or a bowel movement, or after eating a meal. Episodes of dizziness or light-headedness or a syncopal episode always require referral to a physician. Suspect dehydration if the person is on a diuretic or has reduced his or her fluid intake.

Edema (swelling) of the ankles or legs. Swelling of the ankles or legs that can be indented by pressing with the finger can be caused by a number of medical conditions. Common causes include heart failure, venous disease, as well as liver or kidney failure. If of recent onset and associated with pain, it may be due to an infection or a blood clot in one of the veins. If new, painful, unilateral, or progressive, or if it extends above the ankle or there is oozing of fluid, referral to a physician is indicated.

Shortness of breath (dyspnea). Shortness of breath is one of the most common signs of cardiac or respiratory disease. A physician needs to be consulted if it is of recent onset; progressively severe; occurs at night requiring the person to sit or stand for relief; prevents a person from lying flat; or is associated with other symptoms such as wheezing, bloody sputum, or chest pain.

Palpitations. This term refers to an awareness of the heartbeat. Almost always this symptom is associated with a rapid or irregular heartbeat and requires evaluation. If it is recent in onset, fast, or associated with other symptoms such as syncope, feeling of faintness, or chest pain, a referral is urgent.

High blood pressure. An elevated systolic (≥ 140) or diastolic (≥ 90) blood pressure requires medical evaluation and treatment in most older adults. Any pressure > 200 should be referred immediately to a physician.

Low blood pressure. Any systolic pressure < 100 mm Hg, or any drop in systolic blood pressure of > 20 mm Hg when changing position from lying or sitting to standing, could cause syncope, a stroke, a heart attack, or another serious condition. It could be due to dehydration, blood loss, or a medication. This needs to be confirmed immediately with repeated measurements, and the person needs to be referred to a physician.

Signs of respiratory distress. There are a number of signs of respiratory distress that the health care professional should watch for. These include increased respiratory rate, cyanosis, intercostal indrawing, forward leaning posture, and use of accessory muscles.

- Cyanosis is blue skin around the nail beds and lips or elsewhere. It indicates a low oxygen level and therefore a poor respiratory or cardiovascular status. Cyanosis is not always a reliable sign in persons with darker skin color.

- Intercostal indrawing is the observation of intercostal spaces being "sucked" into the chest on inspiration. This is an indication of fatigue of respiratory muscles.

- Forward leaning posture is an attempt to maximize the efficiency of the respiratory system.

- Paradoxical breathing is observed when the abdominal area does not protrude on inspiration and may indicate weakness of the diaphragm, the main muscle of respiration.

Smoking. Smoking is a long-recognized cause of cardiac and pulmonary diseases. Ceasing to smoke even after decades of smoking is to be vigorously encouraged. One benefit, for example, is that the risks of postsurgical complications are reduced even a few months after stopping.

Exercise and education programs. Persons may be triggered for ADL or IADL interventions. [See ADL and IADL CAPs.]. Evidence is accumulating that persons with many cardiovascular, respiratory, and neurological impairments can respond in a safe and efficient manner to training programs that are physiologically based. In addition to exercise, programs for persons with COPD include education, self-management training, and psychological support. The goal of the programs is to improve physical function and endurance and to teach the person to recognize early signs of an exacerbation in order to avoid emergency room and hospital visits.

Additional Resources

American College of Cardiology/American Heart Association Web site for guidelines: www.acc.org

Global Initiative for Chronic Obstructive Lung Disease (GOLD) Web site: www.goldcopd.com/ and more specifically the guidelines www.goldcopd.com/Guidelineitem.asp?l1=2&l2=1&intId=989

Hunt SA, Baker DW, Chin MH, Cinquegrani MP, Feldman AM, Francis GS, Ganiats TG, Goldstein S, Gregoratos G, Jessup ML, Noble RJ, Packer M, Silver MA, Stevenson LW. 2001. ACC/AHA guidelines for the evaluation and management of chronic heart failure in the adult: A report of the American College of Cardiology/American Heart Association Task Force on Practice Guidelines (Committee to Revise the 1995 Guidelines for the Evaluation and Management of Heart Failure).

Miriam Hospital Physical Activity Research Center: www.lifespan.org/behavmed/researchphysical.htm

University of Rhode Island Cancer Prevention Research Center: www.uri.edu/research/cprc/transtheoretical.htm

---

Authors

Iain Carpenter, MD, FRCP
Lewis Lipsitz, MD
Knight Steel, MD

Undernutrition CAP

Problem

The Undernutrition CAP focuses on the nutritional support of adults who are below their "medically recommended" ideal body weight, as measured by a low Body Mass Index. Some persons who are triggered for follow-up will already be significantly underweight and thus undernourished, while other persons will be at risk of undernutrition.

Loss of weight has many causes, including the person's lack of knowledge of how to follow a healthy diet; chewing and swallowing difficulties; need for others to help in feeding; cognitive and communication deficits; medical conditions (for example, muscle problems); appetite problems (for example, premature sensation of being full); mood disorders such as depression, anxiety, and behavior problems; medications; limited food choices; and environmental factors (for example, limited finances or appliances that do not work).

There are a number of adverse consequences of undernutrition, some of which could place the person at risk of premature death. Other consequences include continued weight loss, functional decline, heart problems, skin problems, and risk of infection. At the same time, for persons with terminal or preterminal disease, one needs to consider first the overall care plan. Heroic nutritional interventions at such times may not be desired or appropriate.

Overall Goals of Care

- Address underlying diseases, conditions, or medications that contribute to undernutrition or risk of it, if possible.

- Implement a reasonable treatment plan to ensure adequate caloric intake and thus prevent further weight loss or underweight.

- Increase quality of life by preventing the negative consequences of undernutrition.

Undernutrition CAP Trigger

There are three levels to the Undernutrition CAP trigger, all based on the person's Body Mass Index (BMI), which represents the ratio of the person's weight to height. Thus, the only items required to calculate this trigger are weight and height.

At the same time, this assumes these items have been accurately measured, and the interRAI assessment tools provide a full description of how this is to be accomplished.

TRIGGERED — HIGH RISK

This group includes persons with **both** a baseline BMI score lower than 19 **and** who do not have a clear indication that death is near. Such persons are universally recognized to be underweight.

The BMI can also indicate the extent of undernutrition: a BMI of less than 16 =

---

severely undernourished; a BMI of 16 to 17 = moderately undernourished; and a BMI of 18 = mildly undernourished.

About one-half of the persons in this group will regularly leave 25% or more of their food uneaten, and they will be more likely than others to lose weight in the future.

This group includes about 10% of persons in long-term care facilities and 8% of persons receiving home care.

TRIGGERED — MEDIUM RISK

These persons have **both** a baseline BMI score of 19 to 21 **and** have no clear indication that death is near.

Although not customarily judged to be underweight, about one in five long-term care facility residents in this group will fall into the 18 or lower BMI range by their next full interRAI assessment. Four out of ten of these persons will regularly leave 25% or more of their food uneaten at most meals.

This group includes about 18% of persons in long-term care facilities and 14% of persons receiving home care.

NOT TRIGGERED

All other persons. This group includes about 73% of persons in long-term care facilities and 78% of persons receiving home care.

Undernutrition CAP Guidelines

The following review works through a list of the problems that relate to a person's undernutrition and, as relevant, they should be addressed in the care plan.

First, determine whether the person is leaving a significant amount of food uneaten at most meals. About one-half of those triggered fall into this category. When this is the case, the key to assessment and care is to reverse this situation. Without an active plan to reverse this situation, the vast majority of these persons will continue to leave significant amounts of food uneaten in the future. In comparing those who leave food uneaten with those who do not, higher rates of the following are seen: abnormal laboratory values (70% vs. 40%); a greater likelihood of being on a new drug (60% vs. 30%); having a cardiovascular problem, for example, hypertension (51% vs. 29%), or congestive heart failure (CHF) (23% vs. 10%); and a recent decline in ADLs (31% vs. 10%).

For persons who do not leave food uneaten, the key to assessment is to determine what they are being given to eat. Like all underweight persons, they might benefit from more complex carbohydrates, whole grains, vegetables, fruit, proteins, and in some cases, fat. But this remains a significant challenge for those triggered by this CAP. The key is to get the person to eat more calories (at least 1,600 a day for an average-sized woman and 2,000 a day for a similar man). To do that, there should be a conversation with the person about his or her food preferences and what it would take to begin to increase slowly her or his caloric intake.

Assessment of Current Eating Patterns

Failure to eat food provided at meals. Even a few days of insufficient food intake could lead to a downward process, with accelerated weight loss and de-conditioning. Unfortunately, over 40% of the persons triggered will regularly leave a significant proportion of their meals uneaten. Thus, regularly monitoring food intake is important.

■ Simple monitoring questions: Count the number of meals and between-meal supplements normally provided during the day (for example, one breakfast, lunch, dinner, and all supplements on a given day). What proportion of the food was left uneaten? Is there a pattern as to which foods are left uneaten — for example, meat, potatoes, pasta, bread, vegetables, or fruit? Is the person uninterested in eating processed foods?

- Food offered or available is not congruent with the person's food choices (for example, no meats, flavorless), allergies or food intolerance (for example, not lactose-free), religious tenets, or food quality (for example, not like what spouse used to prepare).

- The intervals between meals, particularly the fasting hours from the last meal in the evening to the first in the morning.

- New medication or treatment regimen that might reduce interest in food. [See Appropriate Medications CAP.]

- Unwilling to accept food supplements or eat more than three meals a day.

- Food not meeting special dietary requirements.

Factors to Be Considered in Altering Current Eating Patterns

Assess the person's food preferences. Include types of foods, types of spices, when he or she likes to eat, and what to avoid.

Swallowing problems (dysphagia). This mechanical problem in swallowing is normally associated with one or more of a number of medical conditions or treatments (for example, esophagitis, injury from radiation, a malignancy in the neck or esophagus, a stroke, Parkinson's disease, a diverticulum or a stricture, a foreign body, or end-stage dementia). If dysphagia is present, consider referral for a swallowing assessment.

- Issues of concern include reluctance to eat certain foods, slowness in eating, complaint of food sticking in the back of the mouth or in the chest, pain on swallowing or when lying down, coughing or choking when eating, and regurgitation of food.

- If on a special diet, could the person eat and swallow without this type of diet? The monotony of such diets can themselves lead to lessened intake.

- If esophagitis is caused by reflux, treating this problem might help to resolve the swallowing problem.

Dental problems. Dental problems might have various causes (for example, a broken or fractured tooth, bleeding gums, loose dentures, oral lesions, dry mouth, or generally poor oral hygiene).

- **Broken or fractured teeth.** Persons with broken teeth require professional attention.

- **Bleeding gums.** Bleeding from around the teeth can be due to inflammation of the gums (gingivitis) or destructive inflammation of the bone surrounding the teeth (periodontitis), and systemic illnesses or medications.

- Attention should be paid to regular procedures in oral hygiene.

- Professional attention is often warranted if bleeding is present.

- **Problems with loose or sore dentures.** Dentures causing soreness need to be evaluated by a dentist to determine whether they can be adjusted or if replacement is necessary.

- **Lip or mouth lesions (cold sores, fever blisters, canker sores, new lumps in mouth).** There are many lesions that occur on the lips and in the mouth that affect chewing. A dentist or physician should evaluate lesions that fail to completely heal within 2 weeks.

■ **Problems with taste or smell.** Older adults frequently complain of difficulties with taste or smell. One of the most common causes is poor oral hygiene.

■ **Dry mouth.** This condition may be caused by multiple medications, diseases, head and neck radiation, and dehydration. The medications commonly implicated include antihypertensives, anxiolytics, antidepressants, antipsychotics, anticholinergics, and antihistamines. [See Medications CAP.]

Need for others to assist in eating. A reduced ability to feed oneself can be due either to cognitive or physical deficits.

■ Cognitive deficits relate to staying focused on the act of eating or an inability to comprehend the sequences needed in eating.

■ Physical deficits include musculoskeletal problems related to conditions such as arthritis, contractures, loss of range of motion in an arm, an inability to sit up, or a missing limb.

Approaches to treatment can involve the support of others, prosthetic strategies, and reconditioning/retraining. Feeding an eating-dependent person can require 30 to 45 minutes. Prosthetic approaches include the use of special equipment (for example, a weighted spoon), provision of foods the person can eat using his or her residual abilities (for example, a texture-modified menu, finger foods). Retraining consideration will require a consult by an occupational therapist.

Disease conditions. Acute and chronic disease, and especially malignancy, can affect the person's nutritional needs by reducing the person's appetite or interest in food or by requiring special feeding or nutritional requirements. Among the conditions and diseases to be considered are

■ Dementia and other neurological diseases, arthritis, asthma, COPD, heart disease, liver disease, renal disease, cancer, diabetes, thyroid disease, or a dental or oral condition.

■ Any recent acute illness or operation can result in weight loss. The problem may be the postoperative course and not the underlying disease itself. Such persons may benefit from a program of adequate nutrition and exercise.

■ Any acute disease or condition including a fever or an infection, and pain, especially gastrointestinal pain.

Cognitive and communication problems. Insufficient food intake and weight loss is associated with the severity of a person's cognitive deficit (especially for a person with a Cognitive Performance Scale [CPS] score of 4 to 6, which translates into a Mini Mental State Examination [MMSE] score of less than 10). [See Cognitive Loss and Communication CAPs.] The mechanisms vary, but can include a decline in cues to feed oneself, to chew, to swallow; a decrease in the pleasure of eating; and the emergence of a variety of disruptive behaviors such as wandering in search of pleasurable foods. Primary intervention strategies could be dictated by these conditions, including nonthreatening approaches to feeding persons who are physically aggressive or the introduction of a prompting schedule to ensure that all or almost all of the food is eaten.

Depression. Depression can cause some persons to decrease the amount of food they eat. A score of 3 or higher on interRAI's Depression Rating Scale (DRS) suggests a possible clinically relevant depression. [See Mood CAP.]

Medications. Adverse drug effects are common reversible causes of decreased nutritional intake. Several drugs have been noted to alter food intake through changes in appetite or the senses of taste and smell, or through adverse gastrointestinal side effects. In addition, drugs may interfere with the absorption, metabolism, and excretion of nutrients. On the other hand, the person's ability to cope with everyday living (such as shopping for food and cooking) can be limited when drugs do not lead to the anticipated relief of symptoms (for example, pain). Hence, the prescribed medications should be reviewed by the physician and, when necessary, changed to other types with fewer side effects.

- Those using the following drugs may require an adjustment of their nutritional care plan: diuretics, certain cardiac drugs, anti-inflammatory drugs, and antiparkinsonian drugs. [See Medications CAPs.]

Need for special diets. Determine which type of special diet the person is on, if any, and whether there is a need to continue that diet. Consult a dietician as needed.

- Diabetic diet and restriction of a variety of foods

- Weight gain diet

- Therapeutic diet — high calorie or high protein diets that have been chopped or blended

The physical and social environment. Normal eating requires more than the serving of complete nutrition. The psychosocial setting must be suitable for the eating experience, including the physical layout and who is in the dining space with the person.

Prospective monitoring:

- Leaving food uneaten

- Continued weight loss

- How well the person uses adaptive equipment

- Continued need for cueing or assistance with eating

- Emergence or continuation of a swallowing problem

- Changes in food preferences

- Assess the "energy density" of the food served

Additional Resource

National Institute for Health and Clinical Excellence Quick Reference Guide. 2006. (February). Oral nutrition support, enteral tube feeding, and parenteral nutrition. www.guideline.gov/summary/summary.aspx?doc_id=8739#s24

Authors
Gunnar Ljunggren, MD, PhD
Harriet Finne-Soveri, MD, PhD
John N. Morris, PhD, MSW

Problem

The Dehydration CAP alerts the care professional to the need to assess for possible dehydration. Normally, the body maintains an appropriate quantity of fluid within its cells and the vascular system. This involves maintaining a balance between the amount of water taken in and the quantity excreted by the kidneys and lost in breathing, sweating, and defecating. Dehydration is a condition where the amount lost exceeds the amount taken in by a person who has the appropriate amount to start with.

A physical examination may provide evidence that the person is dehydrated. However, in older persons, diagnosing dehydration by assessing the degree of tenting of the skin when pinched or the dryness of the mucous parts of the mouth is usually not recommended. Laboratory studies often offer an important indication of the presence of dehydration. In a dehydrated person, the BUN/creatinine ratio in blood almost always increases above approximately 25, and the concentration of hemoglobin in the blood may rise as well. Under most circumstances, the concentration of sodium in the serum rises, as the body usually loses water in excess of salt. If there is a significant degree of dehydration, the person's blood pressure may fall and there may be an associated increase in the pulse rate.

Dehydration is associated with a long list of medical conditions including gastroenteritis, diarrhea, infection, renal disease, and excessive use of diuretics. Older persons may become dehydrated in very hot weather when they do not increase their fluid intake appropriately. Fluids may need to be administered orally or intravenously, depending on the cause of the dehydration and the severity of the condition. Appropriate monitoring of the serum sodium and potassium levels as well as renal function is often required.

Overall Goals of Care

- Identify and treat the underlying cause(s) of dehydration.
- Rehydrate the person, with the course of treatment dependent on the extent of the deficits.
- Establish an appropriate approach to monitoring and laboratory testing to ensure recovery and maintenance of an appropriate fluid balance.
- Prevent associated complications (hypotension, falls, delirium, constipation).
- Provide comfort to those for whom treatment is primarily supportive.

21

This CAP is based on two items in the interRAI assessment instruments: dehydration and insufficient fluid. Both have relatively low prevalence. The rate of dehydration reported on interRAI assessment instruments ranges from less than 1% up to about 5%, while insufficient fluid rates of 3 to 10% are common. When both problems are present, the clinical significance is likely to be more serious. Two trigger levels, high and low, are specified. Persons in the high-level group have one or more obvious causes for or complications of dehydration. Their clinical course mandates immediate review by a physician. Persons in the low-level group, while still requiring close clinical oversight, may be able to be managed by increasing fluid intake and monitoring the person closely.

Over a 90-day period, about one-half of the persons assessed as dehydrated (based on these two items) will typically no longer be assessed as dehydrated. Thus, there are two keys to this CAP. First, be vigilant to ensure that a person with these problems is identified as requiring treatment. Second, intervene to make sure the person is rehydrated properly and his or her associated clinical problems are addressed.

TRIGGERED — HIGH RISK

Persons in this category have first been assessed as dehydrated and/or receiving insufficient fluids. Second, they have been assessed as having one or more of the following causes for or complications of dehydration:

- Diarrhea
- Vomiting
- Delirium (for example, the recent onset of one or more of the following conditions: easily distracted, restlessness, varying mental function, lethargy, disorganized speech, and altered perception)
- Fever
- Dizziness
- Syncope
- Constipation
- Weight loss (5% or more in the last 30 days)

This group includes about 2 to 6% of persons in long-term care facilities, 1% of persons receiving home care, and less than 1% of older adults living independently in the community.

TRIGGERED — LOW RISK

Persons in this category have been assessed as dehydrated and/or receiving insufficient fluids. However, they do **not** have any of the associated conditions noted previously. This group includes about 2% of persons in long-term care facilities, 4% of persons receiving home care, and less than 1% of older adults living independently in the community.

NOT TRIGGERED

All other persons. This group includes about 97% of persons in long-term care facilities, 94% of persons receiving home care, and 99% of older adults living independently in the community.

Identification of the Person's Capacity to Be Involved in His or Her Own Treatment

Many persons triggered by the Dehydration CAP, no matter where they live, will present with a functional or cognitive problem. The first step in designing a care plan is to assess the seriousness of the problem and then the likelihood the person can take a meaningful role in resolving it. For this CAP, it is assumed that such a role can be played when the person has the following three capabilities.

- First, the person has a Cognitive Performance Score of less than 4.
- Second, the person has the ability to move about his or her living space (by walking or in a wheelchair) without the physical help of others and has access to appropriate fluids.
- Third, the person will participate in an appropriate monitoring activity to be sure the dehydration and its cause are adequately addressed.

This definition applies to about 20% of triggered persons in long-term care facilities, 70% of triggered persons receiving home care, and almost all triggered older adults living independently in the community.

Physician Communication and Involvement in Assessing and Care Planning

Initial management. Clinicians must note that the Dehydration CAP has been triggered and assess the person with respect to the degree of dehydration and whether the person has a high- or a low-level trigger for dehydration. When the person has a high-level trigger, an immediate response is warranted. The clinician should communicate these findings to a physician. In addition, factors that may have contributed to or caused dehydration should be brought to the physician's attention. The more comprehensive the information, the easier it will be to determine an appropriate course of action in a timely fashion. For example, knowing that the person has a low-grade fever (which is a high-level trigger feature) and has not been taking fluids well while continuing to take a diuretic will help formulate the course of action.

Clinical Observations (many of which can be drawn from the interRAI Assessment)

Are there signs suggesting the presence of dehydration?

- A rapid pulse or a significant increase in the pulse rate upon assuming an upright position.
- Hypotension, or a change in blood pressure of more than 20 mm Hg upon assuming an upright position.
- Is the person lethargic, confused, or delirious?

Are there signs of an infection?

- Specifically, is there fever, cough, lethargy, dysuria, mental status change, diarrhea, or vomiting?

Changes in the person's oral intake:

- Does the person leave food uneaten, consuming less than 25% of meals?
- Has the person taken in an adequate quantity of fluid?

- Is the person taking an excessive dose of a laxative?
- Does the person have a swallowing problem?
- Does the person tell you that he or she is thirsty?
- Does the person limit the input of fluid due to a fear of incontinence?

Other considerations that may be relevant to dehydration:

- Is the person on a diuretic or has the dose been increased recently?
- Is the person on a fluid restriction?
- Is the person on a newly prescribed diet?
- Is the person on a restricted diet?
- Is an intake and output record kept?
- Does the person have a disease known to increase the likelihood of dehydration?
- Does the person have a history of dehydration?
- Does the person have abdominal pain, with or without diarrhea, nausea, or vomiting?

Illnesses that predispose to limitations in maintaining normal fluid balance:

- Is the person a diabetic, or has there been a change in the medications prescribed for diabetes?
- Does the person have a swallowing problem that limits the ability to increase fluid intake when needed?
- Does the person have a significant degree of renal failure or a known disease of the kidney?
- Is the person lethargic for any reason?
- Is there newly present constipation, fecal impaction, or weight loss?
- Does the person have any behavioral disturbance that precludes him or her from taking sufficient quantities of fluid?
- Is there evidence of a new stroke or recent change in mental status?
- Is the person medically unstable?
- Did the person have a recent acute event, for example, hip surgery, that might predispose to dehydration?
- Has there been a recent decline in ADLs?
- Does the person have a disease, such as Parkinson's disease, that may require an unusually long time to eat?
- Has the person recently stopped taking steroids for any condition? (This may require immediate medical intervention.)

Additional Resources

Fish LC, Davis KM, Minaker KL. 1997. Dehydration. In Morris JN, Lipsitz LA, Murphy KM, Belleville-Taylor P, eds. *Quality care in the nursing home.* St. Louis, MO: Mosby. **Note:** This chapter provides a comprehensive approach to assessment and management of dehydration in the nursing home. Case examples are presented.

Mentes, JC. 1998. *Hydration management research-based protocol.* The University of Iowa Gerontological Nursing Interventions Research Center, Research Dissemination Core. **Note:** This protocol provides helpful information for developing a comprehensive care plan for persons with dehydration. www.nursing.uiowa.edu

Mentes J, Buckwalter K. 1997. Getting back to basics. Managing hydration to prevent acute confusion in frail elders. *Journal of Gerontological Nursing* 23(10): 48–51.

Palmer JB, Drennan JC, Baba M. 2000. Evaluation and treatment of swallowing impairments. *Am Fam Physician* (April 15) 61(8): 2453–62.

Weinburg A, Minaker K, The Council on Scientific Affairs, American Medical Association. 1995. Dehydration: Evaluation and management in older adults. *JAMA* 274: 1552–56.

Weinburg A, Pals J, Levesque P, Beals L, Cunningham T, Minaker K. 1994. Dehydration and death during febrile episodes in the nursing home. *JAGS* 42: 968–71.

Authors

Kenneth L. Minaker, MD
Knight Steel, MD
John N. Morris, PhD, MSW

Feeding Tube CAP

Problem

The Feeding Tube CAP triggers persons with a feeding tube, addressing issues relative to the use of a feeding tube and its potential removal.

The vast majority of feeding tubes in long-term care facilities are percutaneous endoscopic gastrostomy (PEG) tubes — inserted through the stomach wall. Rarely, jejunostomy tubes (J-tubes) are used, which are similar to PEG tubes but are placed beyond the stomach in the gastrointestinal tract, in the jejunum. Both PEG tubes and J-tubes are intended for long-term use (longer than 2 weeks). Nasogastric tubes (NG), which are inserted through a nostril and into the stomach, are intended for short-term acute conditions or as a trial prior to the initiation of long-term feeding (for example, after an acute stroke). These tubes are uncomfortable, may cause nasal and esophageal irritation, and are undignified. Therefore, it is recommended that they not be used for more than 2 weeks. The major focus of this CAP relates to the use of long-term feeding tubes.

There are several causes of eating and swallowing problems among persons in long-term care facilities and those living in the community and receiving home care services. The information presented in this CAP needs to be tailored to the specific clinical considerations in each group and to the broader goals of care of the person (that is, comfort or life prolongation). For example, persons with advanced dementia have an irreversible progressive illness and thus, eating problems need to be considered within the context of end-of-life care. In contrast, dysphagia may be a potentially reversible complication in acute stroke patients, in which case tube-feeding may only be needed temporarily. Persons with Parkinson's disease or other motor neuron diseases may have chronic swallowing problems that require long-term feeding interventions. Finally, head and neck cancers may cause structural complications that result in feeding problems. In all cases, decision making about feeding problems should be shared among practitioners, the person being served, and, when appropriate, family members after considering the particular clinical situation, treatment options, and the person's preferences.

Facts about Tube Feeding

- There is no evidence that the use of a feeding tube improves **survival** in persons with advanced dementia.

- Tube feeding **will not prevent aspiration** of gastric contents or oral secretions. Persons who aspirate prior to the placement of a feeding tube likely will continue to aspirate with the tube.

- The association between the provision of nutrition via feeding tube and the prevention of **pressure ulcers** remains unproven.

- Many family members are concerned that without tube feeding, a terminally ill person will be **hungry or thirsty**. However, it has been shown that persons who are terminally ill do not experience hunger or thirst beyond what can be alleviated with ice chips or glycerin swabs.

Overall Goals of Care

- Ensure that feeding decisions are in accordance with the overriding goals of care.

- Minimize tube feeding in advanced dementia.

- Ensure the person using a feeding tube receives proper care to manage tube feeding, maintains nutrition, and avoids complications.

- Review periodically the appropriateness of the continued use of tube feeding.

- When not appropriate, consider steps to discontinue tube feeding.

Feeding Tube CAP Trigger

All persons with a feeding tube will be triggered for review. However, this group is divided according to their cognitive abilities.

TRIGGERED — HAS SOME RESIDUAL COGNITIVE ABILITIES

This subgroup is defined by two factors:

- The person has a feeding tube.

- The person has at least some ability to engage in everyday decision making (a score from Independent to Moderately Impaired).

This subgroup is more likely to be involved in their own decision making about feeding tube use. They will almost always have at least some ability to understand and be understood by others.

This group includes about 3% of persons in long-term care facilities, 1% of persons receiving home care, and almost no older adults living independently in the community.

TRIGGERED — ABSENCE OF COGNITIVE ABILITIES

This subgroup is defined by two factors:

- The person has a feeding tube.

- The person has no ability to engage in everyday decision making (a score of Severely Impaired to No Discernable Consciousness).

This subgroup includes persons who have profound problems. They have little or no ability to communicate with others. Almost all are functionally dependent in all ADLs (they have an ADL Hierarchy score of 6). Eighty percent or more cannot balance themselves in a sitting position, have a swallowing problem, and have no control over their bladder.

This group includes about 3% of persons in long-term care facilities, 1% of persons receiving home care, and almost no older adults living independently in the community.

NOT TRIGGERED

All other persons (those without a feeding tube). The "Not Triggered" group includes about 94% of persons in long-term care facilities, 98% of persons receiving home care, and all, or almost all, persons living independently in the community.

Involvement of the Health Care Team in the Assessment and Management of Tube-Fed Persons

The use of feeding tubes is a complex issue. The expertise of many disciplines is required to assess and care properly for persons with feeding tubes. Nurses play the primary role and are in the position to identify when the expertise of other team members is needed. Nurses must be prepared to alert the physician and dietician to ongoing care issues, complications, and concerns about the appropriateness of tube feeding. It is recommended that a nutritionist or dietician regularly follow all tube-fed persons to assure appropriate intake corresponds with needs. Other disciplines that may be involved include speech and language pathologists (to assess eating and swallowing capabilities), occupational therapists (for positioning to avoid aspiration), social workers, and clergy (for ethical dilemmas and psychosocial support).

Have psychosocial issues been considered? Eating is an enjoyable social activity, and feeding another person is symbolic of caregiving. Loss of the ability to eat independently can have adverse psychosocial implications for both the person and family members.

- Monitor for signs of depression. [See Mood CAP.]
- Consider other ways to socially engage the person with a feeding tube.
- Provide emotional and social support from social workers, clergy, and other members of the health care team.

Nursing Observations

Provide Ongoing Management of Person with Tube Feed

The DAILY management of a tube-fed person should include the following:

- Clean local area around insertion site.
- Check skin around insertion site for signs of bleeding or local infection (for example, redness, swelling, purulent drainage).
- Monitor for signs or symptoms of gastrointestinal obstruction (abdominal distension, pain, cramping, hard abdomen, loss of bowel sounds, vomiting, high residuals, diarrhea, lack of bowel movements, or fecal impaction).
- Monitor fluid status (dehydration or fluid overload, vomiting).
- Monitor for tube dislodgement.
- Provide nutritional supplements via feeding tube continuously or as boluses several times daily. The choice of nutritional supplement and mode of delivery should be decided by a physician or nutritionist with physician orders.

Periodic evaluations and consultations should include the following:

- Weight checked at least monthly.
- Lab tests performed periodically to monitor electrolytes, serum albumin, and hematocrit.
- Regular periodic evaluations by a nutritionist or dietician.
- Periodic assessment for the possibility of resuming oral feeding. A speech and language pathologist or occupational therapist can help with this assessment.

- Regular changing and replacement of PEG tubes and J-tubes. Individual programs or facilities may differ in their protocol (for example, every 3 months).

Identify and Avoid Complications of Tube-Feeding

Are any of the following direct complications of tube feeding present upon daily evaluation?

Complication	Average % Occurrence	Sign	Actions for Consideration
Infection			
Minor	4	Cellulitis around tube insertion	Local antibiotic ointment
Major	1	Fever, hypotension, diaphoresis (sweating)	Consult physician
Bleeding			
Minor	< 1	Bleeding around insertion	Consult physician
Major	almost 0	Hypotension, drop in Hematocrit, frank blood	Medical emergency; stabilize person and consult physician
Diarrhea and cramping	12	Pain, diarrhea, dehydration	Examine abdomen for signs of obstruction* Consult physician Rule out GI infection Consult nutritionist (may need to change supplement)
Nausea and vomiting	9	Nausea, vomiting, abdominal distention, dehydration	Check for residuals,* slow feeds,* examine abdomen for signs of obstruction,* avoid aspiration Consult physician and nutritionist
Minor tube problem	4		All may require physician consultation
Dislodgement		Tube no longer in place	Replace tube (Foley catheter sometimes used)
Blockage		Disrupted flow of supplement	Flush tube with water or ginger ale
Leakage		Leaking around tube	Tube may need replacing (Foley catheter sometimes used)
Major tube problem (Bowel perforation)	< 1	Absent bowel sounds, tense abdomen, nausea, vomiting, diarrhea, or absent bowel movements (fecal impaction), hypotension	Medical emergency Consult physician immediately

*Definitions:
Signs of obstruction: Include abdominal cramps, vomiting, abdominal distention, absent or high-pitched bowel sounds, abdominal tenderness.
Residuals: The amount of food remaining in the stomach upon gastric aspiration prior to giving a feeding.
Slow feeding: Feeding that progresses slower than the prescribed drip rate.

Are any of the following other serious complications related to the use of feeding tubes present?

- **Aspiration** — Tube feeding will not prevent a person from aspirating. Persons who were aspirating prior to the feeding tube insertion remain at high risk of recurrent aspiration of oral secretions and gastric contents. Silent aspiration occurs often. Aspiration is uncomfortable for the person and can lead to aspiration pneumonia.

- **Strategies to prevent aspiration in a tube-fed person include the following:**
  - Choose appropriate rate for tube feeding (consult with physician and nutritionist/dietician)
  - Monitor for high residuals
  - Oral suctioning when appropriate
  - If taking food orally, use proper feeding techniques. Consult nutritionist, occupational therapist, or speech and language pathologist, as necessary

- **Signs and symptoms of aspiration pneumonia:**
  - Coughing, shortness of breath, increased sputum production
  - Fever, increased respiratory rate, diaphoresis, decline in mental status, agitation
  - Hypotension, signs of dehydration

- **Laboratory results:**
  - Elevated white blood cell count, elevated blood urea nitrogen, creatinine, or sodium
  - Consolidation on chest x-ray
  - Hypoxia

- **Actions for consideration:**
  - Stabilize person (for example, consider the use of oxygen)
  - Consult physician, respiratory therapist
  - Person may need antibiotics and parenteral IV hydration

Is the person physically restrained or receiving psychotropic medication? Persons who are tube fed often have cognitive problems and are easily agitated. They may try to pull out the feeding tube. Thus, agitated persons with feeding tubes are at high risk of being restrained or given psychotropic medications for sedation. Studies have shown that persons who live in long-term care facilities who are tube fed are more likely to be restrained compared to those who are not tube fed. **Both physical restraints and psychotropic medications can have serious adverse consequences and should be avoided and used only as a last resort to maintain the tube.** [See CAPs on Physical Restraints and Appropriate Medications.]

Periodically assess the appropriateness of ongoing tube feeding. The decision to insert a feeding tube was made at some prior time. [See CAPs for Undernutrition and Dehydration.] As with all medical therapies, its continued use should be reassessed periodically to ensure that it continues to meet the goals of care for this person. Technically, it is very easy to stop tube feeding (most PEG tubes are designed to be removed with moderate traction safely and painlessly). However, emotionally and ethically, discontinuation of tube feeding can be very difficult, and any psychosocial needs of the person and family should be supported.

Reasons to discontinue tube feeding include the following:

- The person has improved enough to eat and drink by mouth. Consider involving a nutritionist, speech and language pathologist, or occupational therapist in this assessment.

- The person has not improved in overall status or adequate oral intake and tube feeding no longer meets the goals of care. Alternative management strategies to consider include

- A conscientious approach to hand-feeding. While hand-feeding may not provide caloric intake, it may provide some positive quality of life for the person.

- Supportive care (for example, pain control, treatment for shortness of breath, use of glycerin swabs or ice chips to keep the mouth moist, skin care, psychosocial support, etc.) in a terminally ill person.

Steps to Consider in Discontinuation of Tube Feeding in Persons Who Have Not Improved in Swallowing or Adequate Oral Intake

> **Laws must be taken into account with regard to the discontinuation of tube feeding and may differ from jurisdiction to jurisdiction.**

Is the person cognitively intact and capable of making his or her own health care decisions?

- Consider meeting with involved members of the health care team to establish the person's status with regard to tube feeding.

- Consider designating members of the health care team, including the physician, to approach the person to review his or her status, the risks and benefits of tube feeding versus supportive care or hand feeding, and to elicit the person's preference for tube feeding. This must be an **informed** decision.

- Involve a family member(s) in the decision-making process as appropriate.

- Respect the person's choice.

Is the person cognitively impaired and incapable of making his or her own health care decisions?

- Consider meeting with involved members of the health care team to establish the person's status with regard to tube feeding.

- Identify the person who has been either formally or informally designated the substitute decision maker for the person (health care proxy).

- Consider a meeting with the designated members of the health care team, including the physician and the substitute decision maker, to review the person's status, the risks and benefits of tube feeding versus supportive care, and to provide counseling regarding the continuation of tube feeding.

If the person is cognitively impaired and incapable of making his or her own health care decisions, has a substitute decision maker been counseled to consider the following?

- Does the person have a written advance directive indicating whether or not he or she would want to be tube fed in the current situation?

- Has the person ever verbally communicated with family members or health practitioners if he or she would want to be tube fed under the current circumstances?

- After considering what is known about the person's values and preferences, does the substitute decision maker feel the person would want to continue tube feeding in the current situation if the person were capable of making a decision (a substituted judgment)?

- After being informed of the risks and benefits of tube feeding, is it in the person's best interests to continue tube feeding?

Is there conflict between the person's advance directive or best interests and the substitute decision maker's choice?

- In most instances, when the substitute decision maker's choice is fully informed, the choice of the substitute decision maker and the wishes of the person as expressed in the advance directive are the same. In this situation the choice of the substitute decision maker should be respected.

- Rarely, the substitute decision maker's choice may appear to contradict a person's advance directive or best interests. All attempts should be made by the health care team to reach an informed decision with the substitute decision maker. In extraordinary circumstances, referral to an ethics committee or a court may be indicated.

Additional Resources

Finucane TE, Christmas C, Travis K. 1999. Tube feeding in patients with advanced dementia: A review of the evidence. *JAMA* 282: 1365–70. **Note:** This article reviews the current evidence of the impact of tube feeding in patients with advanced dementia.

Gillick MR. 2000. Rethinking the role of tube feeding in patients with advanced dementia. *NEJM* 342: 206–10. **Note:** This thoughtful piece presents the controversies related to tube feeding in advanced dementia.

Mitchell SL, Tetroe A, O'Connor AM. 2000. Making choices: Long-term feeding tube placement in elderly patients. **Note:** This is a booklet and audiotape designed to assist substitute decision makers with the dilemma of whether to place a feeding tube on an older person with eating problems. It contains information regarding tube feeding, including its risks and benefits, substitute decision making, and how to weigh the information together with the patients' values and preferences. The decision aid can be viewed and ordered online at www.lri.ca/programs/ceu/ohdec/decision_aids.htm or by calling the toll free number (U.S. and Canada only) 888-240-7002.

Schneider SM, Raina C, Pugliese P, Pouget I, Rampal P, Hebuterne X. 2001. Outcome of patients treated with home enteral nutrition. *JPEN J Parenter Enteral Nutr.* (July–August) 25(4): 203–9. **Note:** This article is evidence-based and gives additional values to the topics.

Sheehan MN, Belleville-Taylor P, Fiatarone M, Hartery S. 1997. Feeding tubes. In Morris JN, Lipsitz LA, Murphy KM, Belleville-Taylor P, eds. *Quality care in the nursing home.* St. Louis, MO: Mosby. **Note:** This chapter provides a detailed overview of assessment and management of the person with a feeding tube. Case examples are presented.

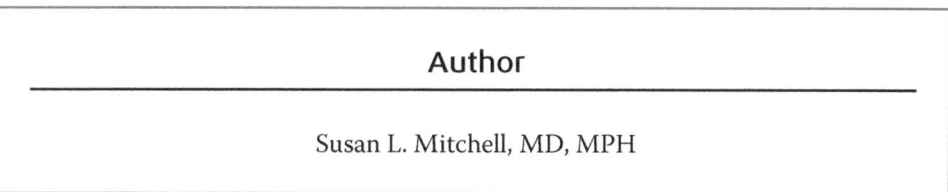

Author
Susan L. Mitchell, MD, MPH

Prevention CAP

Problem

It is preferable to prevent illnesses and disabilities rather than be required to address them once they have occurred. Therefore, the Prevention CAP is designed to alert the health care worker to the need to determine if the person has unmet preventive health requirements (for example, blood pressure screening, immunizations, mammograms) and to meet as many of them as possible in all settings of care. Although preventive health directives often may best be instituted before age 65, there is increasing evidence that many can be introduced profitably even in the later years of life. Some recommendations are designed specifically for use in that time period. It has been suggested that the most reasonable approach to screening most adults, and especially older adults, would be to incorporate such activities into the routine physician visit.

In general, preventive health measures include immunizations and screening for unrecognized health problems. While immunizations are designed to prevent illness, screening is designed to detect unrecognized illness at an early and treatable stage. The goal of both is to reduce morbidity and mortality. Although the advantage of any preventive health intervention is likely to decline with advancing age if measured in years of morbidity saved, prevention is still of great value for most older persons. It must be appreciated that the average 65-year-old currently has a life expectancy approaching 20 years. Furthermore, although many disorders of older adults are chronic and not curable, early detection and treatment of problems that interfere with functioning may result in functional deficits being postponed or even prevented altogether.

Overall Goal of Care

- Ensure that persons who have not received preventive measures are identified and appropriate action is taken.

Prevention CAP Trigger

TRIGGERED BECAUSE PREVENTIVE STRATEGY WAS NOT PURSUED, DESPITE A RECENT PHYSICIAN VISIT

This group includes persons who have recently seen a physician and have not followed one or more of the following prevention strategies:

- Blood pressure measured in the last year

- Colonoscopy test in the last 5 years

- Dental exam in the last year

- Eye exam in the last year

- Hearing exam in the last 2 years

- Influenza vaccine in the last year

- Mammogram in the last 2 years (for women only)
- Pneumovax vaccine in the last 5 years

This triggered group includes about 40% of persons receiving home care and 80% of persons in long-term care facilities.

TRIGGERED BECAUSE PREVENTIVE STRATEGY WAS NOT PURSUED AND THERE HAS BEEN NO RECENT PHYSICIAN VISIT

This group includes persons who have **not** recently seen a physician and have **not** followed one or more of the following prevention strategies:

- Blood pressure measured in the last year
- Colonoscopy test in the last 5 years
- Dental exam in the last year
- Eye exam in the last year
- Hearing exam in the last 2 years
- Influenza vaccine in the last year
- Mammogram in the last 2 years (for women only)
- Pneumovax vaccine in the last 5 years

This triggered group includes 35% of persons receiving home care and almost no persons living in long-term care facilities.

NOT TRIGGERED   This group includes all other persons. The "Not Triggered" group includes about 20% of persons in long-term care facilities and 25% of persons receiving home care.

Prevention CAP Guidelines

The Prevention CAP concept of prevention encompasses a wide variety of tests, procedures, and clinical interventions. This CAP concentrates on some of the more traditional preventive health measures. Many other CAPs relate to prevention of a variety of other problems.

A negative response to any item noted in this CAP raises the possibility of poor preventive health care and further suggests the need to determine whether the person has access to high-quality comprehensive medical care. Persons who have not had specific preventive health tests likely should be recommended for consideration of those tests. The potential benefit and harm derived from each screening procedure and possible intervention must be considered in light of the age and frailty of the person.

The vaccines and screening procedures commonly recommended in the care of adults, and especially older adults, are noted in the following sections. In general, this CAP does not address preventive health measures that require the collection of laboratory data although, unquestionably, the comprehensive management of all older persons requires routinely obtaining some laboratory data both for screening and for establishing a "baseline" for future comparisons. There are considerable data about, but not absolute agreement on, which tests are indicated at what age. Preventive health measures likely to be included in other CAPs are not considered here (for example, items that are pertinent to the prevention of pressure ulcers or the problems related to alcohol consumption).

It is important to note that recommendations for "routine" screening vary among countries. This CAP is based on commonly adopted strategies in many countries. It is important to understand which of these strategies have been adopted in your country, as it may not be possible to implement recommendations without financial support from a government or other relevant funding agency. The country-specific guidelines cited in this CAP are intended to illustrate guidelines that may be found in other countries.

Vaccinations. Older adults especially are susceptible to a number of infectious diseases, in particular those of the lower respiratory tract. Influenza and pneumonia remain the fifth leading cause of death in this age group. The merits of screening older adults to determine if they have received appropriate vaccines are clear. If an older person is admitted to the hospital in the United States for community acquired pneumonia, screening for a history of having received influenza and pneumonia vaccine is the standard of care as determined by Medicare. The Public Health Agency of Canada recommends influenza immunization yearly as well as timely pneumococcal vaccinations for those age 65 and over. If the person has not received these vaccines within the designated time period, they should be offered to the person while in the acute-care setting.

Influenza. Influenza epidemics usually occur in the late fall and winter season, and all older persons should be vaccinated each year before the influenza season except under unusual circumstances (for example, allergy to the vaccine). Because the virus changes on an annual basis, vaccination in one year is not likely to provide significant protection in subsequent years.

The Centers for Disease Control and Prevention (CDC) in the United States recommends this immunization program for all persons 50 years of age and over as well as certain other groups unless there is a specific contraindication. Recently the vaccine has been recommended for many more individuals in other age groups. Similar recommendations are made by the National Advisory Committee on Immunization (NACI) (www.hc-sc.gc.ca). Influenza vaccination is one of the most cost-effective medical interventions available. Of note, older adults have higher hospitalization and death rates from influenza than any other segment of the population and account for 80 to 90% of all influenza-related deaths. Although there is considerable year-to-year variation, vaccines have been shown to be on average 70% effective in preventing influenza, with the remaining 30% often having milder illness than unvaccinated persons.

Pneumococcal disease and other infectious diseases. An immunization program for pneumococcal disease is recommended for almost all older persons. However, it is not given annually. Unless there is a specific contraindication, tetanus immunization every 10 years is recommended for all adult age groups by agencies like the CDC and NACI. Details of immunization programs for other infections, such as hepatitis, varicella, and meningococcal disease, are available on the CDC Web site (www.cdc.gov) or Canadian Immunization Guide (www.phac-aspc.gc.ca/publicat/cig-gci/index-eng.php).

Screening. Traditional screening measures are valuable in circumstances where the disease in question has a high incidence rate and a treatment and/or therapy exists that can cure it or favorably modify its progression if found early. Also, there must be a reasonable likelihood that the person will live and function well for a period of time.

Hypertension. Hypertension is defined as a blood pressure of 140/90, with a systolic pressure of 120 to139 and a diastolic pressure of 80 to 89 viewed as "prehypertensive." Hypertension is a very significant risk factor for both coronary artery disease and cerebrovascular disease.

According to the Joint National Committee on Prevention, Detection, Evaluation and Treatment of High Blood Pressure of the National Institutes of Health (NIH), as many as 90% of persons who are normotensive (having normal blood pressure) at age 55 will develop hypertension over the course of their lives. There is now compelling evidence that lowering blood pressure (including isolated systolic hypertension) is advantageous well into the later years. Several major studies have demonstrated good outcomes when hypertension was controlled, including a reduced incidence of stroke, congestive heart failure, and mortality. Therefore, screening at regular intervals is highly recommended. The level to which the blood pressure should be lowered varies to some degree according to the age of the person and his or her medical conditions.

Recommendations for frequency of screening vary by organization. The Institute of Medicine in the United States suggests that persons age 50 and older without known cardiovascular disease and with a history of normal blood pressure readings should have their blood pressure checked once every 2 years if there are no known risk factors (see also the Canadian Hypertension 2007 Educational Program: www.hypertension.ca/bpc/wp-content/uploads/2008/02/2008publicrecommenda tions.pdf). Most professional organizations would recommend that the blood pressure be measured routinely when adults seek care for most conditions. The proper means of taking the blood pressure can be found on the NIH Web site (www.nih .gov).

Breast cancer. Breast cancer is the most common cancer in women (except for skin cancers). Approximately one in nine women will develop breast cancer. Several factors are associated with a higher risk, such as a mother or sister having breast cancer, as well as the presence of certain genetic markers. There is evidence that breast cancer screening by means of mammography reduces mortality from breast cancer for women over 50 years of age. Of note, newer radiologic and imaging procedures may well be far more effective, but good data are not readily available at this time.

The U.S. Preventive Services Task Force recommends screening mammography, with or without a clinical breast examination, every 1 to 2 years for women age 40 or older. According to the Canadian Task Force on the Periodic Health Examination (CTPHE), women age 50 to 69 should receive screening with clinical breast examination (CBE) and mammography annually. In the United Kingdom, the NHS Breast Screening Programme suggests screening every 3 years for this age group, and it also offers screening to women over 70 at their request.

For women with a strong family history of breast cancer, the age to begin screening and the frequency to do so may be different. The value of the breast self-examination is not clear, and therefore many organizations make no specific recommendation. Data to support formal recommendations about mammography for those above about age 75 to 80 are hard to come by. Screening recommendations must be made in light of the woman's other medical conditions, insofar as they have an impact on her life expectancy. In general, if a woman has a life expectancy of greater than about 6 years, a case can be made to recommend mammography and perhaps newer screening procedures. Many groups recommend that a primary care provider perform breast examinations routinely on their female patients, although data to support the efficacy of this recommendation as a screening measure are lacking.

Colorectal cancer. The lifetime probability that a person will develop colorectal cancer is reported to be about 6 per 100 individuals. There are certain medical conditions that increase the risk. Race-specific rates suggest there are significant genetic factors that increase the incidence of this type of tumor, and certain races appear to have a higher risk of developing colon cancer at a younger age than others. Furthermore, the prevalence of colon cancer varies strikingly around the world, likely in part as a result of different dietary habits and perhaps other environmental factors. In general, the incidence increases with age. In Canada, colorectal cancer is the second most diagnosed cancer in women and third most in males (www .cancercare.on.ca).

Traditional screening tests have included the digital rectal exam and the fecal occult blood test. Regrettably, the evidence that they are valuable screening tools is limited at best. Nonetheless, because of the ease with which they can be carried out, they may be of some value in situations where screening by means of colonoscopy is not available. There are a large number of false positive and false negative tests with the fecal occult blood test. Flexible colonoscopy has become the standard in prevention. In no small part this is because most malignancies of the colon arise from other growths, usually adenomas (benign tumors that have a glandular origin), which can be found and removed by means of this procedure. Other radiologic screening tools are being developed. Of course, should a growth be discovered, likely a colonoscopy will be necessary for biopsy and/or removal. The frequency that a colonoscopy should be performed is under continual review and depends in part on whether or not a polyp (abnormal growth of tissue [tumor] projecting from a mucous membrane) is found on an initial study. Also, some premalignant growths are not easily seen unless the bowel is well cleaned out. It is known that the risks of colonoscopy are greater in the very elderly, and that although the prevalence of colonic neoplasia is higher among older persons, the mean extension in life expectancy is lower among adults age 80 and older compared with those age 50 to 54.

Gynecological (cervical/uterus) cancer. Although some groups have recommended a Pap smear every 1 to 3 years for older women, the upper age limit for screening remains a point of debate. If a woman has been screened regularly and if she does not have a high number of sex partners, the value of continuing screening beyond age 65 appears to be small, assuming she is asymptomatic and has no menstrual bleeding.

Prostate cancer. Although some groups continue to recommend yearly rectal examinations, many leading agencies do not. Screening by means of a PSA test is widely carried out in many places; however, its value as a screening tool remains controversial, in part because of the large number of false positive and false negative tests. However, it has great value in follow-up of men who have been diagnosed with cancer of the prostate.

Sensory impairments. Many preventive strategies involving screening for early hearing loss are addressed in the Communication CAP. It is clear that the provision of hearing aids as well as other assistive devices may produce dramatic improvement in function. With respect to vision, many groups recommend an annual ophthalmologic evaluation in older persons.

Osteoporosis. Approximately 20 to 25 million Americans are at increased risk for fractures because of low bone density. More than one million fractures in the United States each year can be attributed to this condition. According to the Public Health Agency of Canada, about one out of four women and one out of eight men over age 50 have osteoporosis. Similar data are available for other nations, especially those with large numbers of Caucasian women and those in Northern Europe, where decreased exposure to sunlight over long periods of the year results in the limited bio-availability of vitamin D. This issue is addressed in the Falls and Nutrition CAPs.

At this time, screening by means of bone mineral density (BMD) x-rays (test that measures the density of minerals such as calcium to estimate the strength of bones) is recommended for all women age 65 and older by the National Osteoporosis Foundation (www.nof.org). Because such studies measure bone density and not bone structure itself, these recommendations may be modified in the near future when other screening mechanisms become widely available. Screening recommendations for men are under consideration.

Skin testing for tuberculosis. In the United States, skin testing for tuberculosis is now a two-step process. If the initial PPD (Purified Protein Derivative TB Skin Test or Mantoux) is negative, a repeat study is recommended usually in about 2 weeks.

Screening blood tests. There are a large number of screening blood tests that can be and often are used in different age groups. The merits of each test individually are difficult to ascertain. This should not be construed to mean that there is no merit in doing any number of blood tests, for example the measurement of hemoglobin, B12 levels, and thyroid function, on a regular basis. It is unclear how frequently they should be ordered. Screening for the various lipid abnormalities, especially in men beginning at age 40 and in women perhaps at a somewhat older age, is recommended by many professional organizations.

Smoking. Smoking is hazardous at any age both to those who smoke and those in the environment of the smoker. In addition, there is evidence that ceasing to smoke even a few weeks prior to an elective surgical procedure will decrease the risk of some of the complications associated with that procedure. The Center for Medicare and Medicaid Services (CMS) in the United States requires all persons admitted with a diagnosis of pneumonia to an acute-care facility to be screened for smoking and to be given smoking cessation material if the person does smoke.

Miscellaneous. The value of screening for certain tumors, specifically ovarian cancer (for example, by means of serum tumor markers, ultrasound), lung cancer (chest x-ray, sputum cytology), and cardiac disease (by means of CT scanning) is not clear at this time. Recently there has been a recommendation to screen men age 65 and above for presence of abdominal aortic aneurysm. If normal, no further screening is recommended at this time.

Lastly, screening to determine if there is a need to counsel a person about the value of an exercise program targeted to his or her clinical condition is strongly recommended by most.

Additional Resources

Fact sheets on immunization developed by Victoria, Australia, Department of Human Services: www.health.vic.gov.au/immunisation/factsheets
Health Canada Web site: www.hc-sc.gc.ca
NHS Breast Screening fact sheet: www.cancerscreening.nhs.uk/breastscreen/publications/over70.pdf
Osteoporosis Canada Web site: www.osteoporosis.ca
U.S. Joint National Committee on Prevention, Detection, Evaluation, and Treatment of High Blood Pressure: www.nhlbi.nih.gov/guidelines/hypertension/jnc7full.pdf

---

Authors

Knight Steel, MD
John P. Hirdes, PhD

Appropriate Medications CAP

Problem

Changes associated with aging affect an individual's capacity to benefit from and tolerate medications (drugs), and inappropriate use of medications can prove harmful to the person. Age-associated changes occur in the absorption, distribution, metabolism, and excretion of many medications due to physiological changes at the organ and cellular level, particularly in the kidneys and gastrointestinal tract. These changes predispose the aging person to adverse effects from many medications. Age-related changes in the body composition, notably changes in the proportion of body fat and water, may alter the effects of fat-soluble medications. The older person often has multiple chronic diseases that may further impair not only the pharmacokinetics of drugs, but also their pharmacodynamic effects. Older persons are at particular risk of adverse effects because most take multiple medications.

On the other hand, evidence supports the use of medications in even very old persons as long as there is a significant likelihood of a benefit balanced against the risk and a proper indication for the use of each drug. The dosage of each medication must be appropriate and there must be an appreciation of the possibility of interactions amongst the medications.

Inappropriate medication prescribing for older persons comes in several varieties, including prescribing medications not suitable for older and frail persons, combinations of medications that interact with one another, and medications at doses that are too high for older persons.

Appropriate prescribing includes a process for monitoring the effects of each medication individually and in combination with others being taken, discontinuing the medication after the intended indication for use no longer exists, and at the same time, prescribing a medication when the potential benefit clearly exceeds the risk. **Multiple medications may be necessary and of benefit when the aim is to control multiple chronic illnesses. However, frequent hospitalizations, multiple treating physicians, and the use of over-the-counter medications make the need for frequent periodic review essential.**

In addition to the side effects of each individual medication and the combination of two or more medications being taken, the negative consequences associated with medications include a variety of events, such as the exacerbation of an existing disease, a decline in cognitive or functional capacity, a negative impact on quality of life, as well as an unnecessary use of health services and the associated costs.

Overall Goals of Care

- Promote the proper management of each person, neither overtreating nor undertreating each disease.

- Promote the appropriate dose, timing, and length of use of each drug.

- Promote the ability and desire of each person to adhere to the schedule of medications as prescribed.

(continued)

- Demonstrate the value of monitoring the status of each person and assessing the potential hazards of each medication and helping caregivers recognize an adverse effect as soon as possible.

- Encourage the undertaking of a regular review of the drug regimen

Medications CAP Trigger

TRIGGERED — HIGH PRIORITY

High priority triggers identify persons with nine or more medications, and those with two or more of the conditions listed below. This group contains up to 40% of those in a long-term care facility, a similar percentage of those receiving home care services, and 5 to10% of older persons living in the community.

Both of the following should be present:

- Nine or more medications

- Has two or more of the following conditions:

    - Chest pain

    - Dizziness

    - Edema

    - Shortness of breath

    - Poor health

    - Recent deterioration

NOT TRIGGERED

All other persons.

Note: if any of the following are present, consider completing a medication review:

- Fatigue

- Depression

- Delirium

- Recent cognitive decline

- Fall

- Nausea

- Recent hospitalization

- Weight loss

- Loss of appetite

- Nonspecific complaints such as "I don't feel well" or "I am not myself"

Medications CAP Guidelines

The Medications CAP can be used as a helpful tool for assessing a person's medications. The triggered persons, however, are those who receive nine drugs or more or who have two or more of the conditions noted under "Triggered – High Priority."

Multiple physician prescriptions. To begin, it is important to recognize that more than one physician often may have prescribed the medications taken by the person. In addition, other medications including "natural substances" may be purchased over the counter by the person or a caregiver. All medications should be administered as ordered by the physician. If there are variations, the physician should be informed. The nurse is in the key position to observe or hear directly from the older person or his or her caregivers about signs and symptoms that may be caused by medications — a single drug or a combination of drugs.

Some of the most frequent adverse effects include those in different organ systems:

- Central nervous system — for example, delirium, memory problems, fatigue, depression, tremor

- Cardiovascular — for example, hypotension, dizziness, arrhythmias

- Gastrointestinal — for example, loss of appetite, weight loss, constipation, diarrhea, nausea, vomiting, bleeding

- Urinary tract — for example, incontinence, urinary retention

- Musculoskeletal and trauma — for example, accidents, falls, fractures, decline in functional status

- Pulmonary — for example, wheezing, shortness of breath

- Skin — for example, itching, rash, swelling

When such symptoms are noted, the possibility of a medication causing the symptom should be considered.

The following situations require frequent monitoring and notification of the physician:

- Recent change in cognition [Also see Delirium, Cognitive Loss, and Mood CAPs.]

- Recent change in functional capacity [Also see ADL CAP.]

- Weight loss or gain [See Undernutrition CAP.]

- Recent change in continence [See Urinary Incontinence CAP.]

- Recurrent traumatic event [See Falls CAP.]

- Hospitalization

- The appearance of a new symptom

Some drugs that need particular attention are often (appropriately) used in older persons. To avoid potential adverse events and interactions, it is necessary to review the medications more often in these cases. For example, the following medications require frequent monitoring, especially when initially started:

- Anticoagulants such as warfarin

- Diuretics

- Digoxin

- Antihypertensives

Some medications should be avoided if other options are available. For example, nonsteroidal anti-inflammatory drugs (NSAIDs) carry a risk of gastrointestinal bleeding.

The use of any psychotropic medication requires a proper indication and monitoring over time. [See Behavior CAP.] Medications with anxiolytic, sedative, and hypnotic effects should be used in the lowest possible dose. In addition, these medications should be prescribed for the shortest possible time.

The aim of the medication regimen is to achieve the desired outcome with the fewest medications and the lowest possible dosages. However, the use of multiple medications may often be indicated.

Multiple Medications

Examples of potentially APPROPRIATE polypharmacy:

- Persons with diabetes may be prescribed several types of insulin in addition to oral medications. In addition, cholesterol or blood pressure lowering agents may be needed.

- Persons with a history of a myocardial infarction, congestive heart failure, or hypertension often require several medications.

- Persons with Parkinson's disease often receive multiple medications.

Examples of potentially DANGEROUS situations:

- Persons may be taking the same pharmaceutical agent under two different trade names.

- Persons may be taking a medication for a problem when a nonpharmacological intervention might be of equal or greater benefit.

Some of the most often seen and potentially (but not always) hazardous combinations of drugs include:

- warfarin and a long list of medications

- potassium sparing diuretic and potassium containing medication

---

The physician should be informed when a drug, prescribed on a PRN basis, has not been needed for a significant time. On the other hand, some symptoms, such as pain in a severely ill person, may be undertreated and require an increase in the dose or frequency of administration of the medication or a different pharmaceutical altogether. [See Pain CAP.]

Medication prescribing recommendations derived from clinical practice guidelines have frequently been designed for younger persons with a single chronic condition. When used for older persons with multiple illnesses, they should be reviewed carefully.

An appropriate medication regimen in older persons taking even a single medication, but particularly those taking multiple medications, is presented as a guideline to facilitate the learning process:

- Medication prescription is based on a person's unique needs (indication) and care preferences, and that person's life expectancy as documented in the medical record.

- The potential benefit of a medication should outweigh the risk of its use. Any combination of medications should provide potentially greater benefit than any of its components alone.

- In most circumstances, an agreement with the older person, or his or her informal caregiver, should be sought and the care preferences of the person explored as to the need for every new medication and duration of the treatment.

- The person, or the formal and informal caregivers, should be provided with information about the dosage and schedule of the medication, how soon the expected effect will appear, and what adverse effects might be seen. There must be a specific measurable goal for each medication, and there should be a monitoring plan that may result in a change in the goal or the medication.

- Most medications for older persons should be started with a low dose, with the dose increased until the expected effect is reached **or** an adverse effect is noted. "Start low, go slow."

- The effects of the medication (desired and/or undesired) should be documented regularly by the appropriate health care professional.

- If a medication is discontinued, the condition of the person should be monitored and documented over time.

- Many long-acting medications used for anxiety, for example, should be avoided under most circumstances.

- A medication error or nonadherence to a prescribed regimen requires that the physician be notified.

- A list of medications should include all prescribed medications, over-the-counter medications, and all preparations not classified as medications that have a potential effect on other medications being taken or on the person's condition. This list should be provided to all physicians caring for the person, including consultants.

Contact the physician if questions about medications arise. The nursing staff may help inform the person and/or his or her caregivers about the effects of the medications and the care plan. The nursing staff is in a key position to monitor any clinical changes associated with a change in medications.

Some drug-related conditions and symptoms can be detected by systematic monitoring. This may be deemed appropriate over an agreed period of time, for example 3, 7, or 14 days. Symptoms may best be documented according to time of the day, thereby demonstrating a relationship to a medication. Such systematic monitoring may also suggest the need for a new medication.

Disclaimer: This CAP is not intended to be an all-inclusive guide to medication management. A nurse should always contact a physician if there is any indication of an unexpected medication-related symptom or indeed a change in the clinical situation.

Additional Resources

Boyd CM, Darer J, Boult C, Fried LP, Boult L, Wu AW. 2005. Clinical practice guidelines and quality of care for older patients with multiple comorbid diseases: Implications for pay for performance. *JAMA* 294: 716–24.

Doshi JA, Schaffer T, Briesacher BA. 2005. National estimates of medication use in nursing homes: Findings from the 1997 Medicare current beneficiary survey and the 1996 medical expenditure survey. *JAGS* 53: 438–43.

Fialová D, Topinková E, Gambassi G, Finne-Soveri H, Jónsson PV, Carpenter I, Schroll M, Onder G, Sørbye LW, Wagner C, Reissigová J, Bernabei R for AdHOC project research group. 2005. Potentially inappropriate medication use among home care elderly patients in Europe. *JAMA* 293: 1348–58.

Fick DM, Cooper JW, Wade WE, Waller JL, Maclean JR, Beers MH. 2003. Updating the Beers criteria for potentially inappropriate medication use in older adults. *Arch Intern Med.* 163: 2716–24.

Gandhi TK, Weingart SN, Borus J, Seger AC, Peterson J, Burdick E, Seger DL, Shu K, Frederico F, Leape LL, Bates DW. 2003. Adverse drug effects in ambulatory care. *NEJM* 348(16): 1556–64.

Knight EL, Avorn J. 2001. Quality indicators for appropriate medication use in vulnerable elders. *Ann Intern Med* 135(8S): 703–10.

Lane CJ, Bronskill SE, Sykora K, Dhalla IA, Anderson GM, Mamdani MM, Gill SS, Gurwitz JH, Rochon PA. 2004. Potentially inappropriate prescribing in Ontario community-dwelling older adults and nursing home residents. *JAGS* 52: 861–66.

McLeod PJ, Huang AR, Tamblyn RM, Gayton DC. 1997. Defining inappropriate practices in prescribing for elderly people: A national consensus panel. *CMAJ* 156: 385–91.

Monastero R, Palmer K, Qiu C, Winblad B, Fratiglioni L. 2007. Heterogeneity in risk factors for cognitive impairment, no dementia: Population-based longitudinal study from the Kungsholmen project. *AM J Geriatr Psychiatry* 15(1): 60–69.

Redelmeier DA, Tan SH, Booth GL. 1998. The treatment of unrelated disorders in patients with chronic medical diseases. *NEJM* 338: 1516–20.

Simon SR, Chan KA, Soumerai SB, Wagner AK, Andrade SE, Feldstein AC, Lafata JE, Davis RL, Gurwitz JH. 2005. Potentially inappropriate medication use by elderly persons in U.S. health maintenance organizations, 2000–2001. *JAGS* 53: 227–32.

Socialstyrelsen. 2003. Indikatorer för utvärdering av kvaliteten i äldres läkemedelsterapi. Socialstyrelsens förslag. Artikelnummer: 110–20.

Veehof LJG, Stewart RE, Haaijer-Ruskamp FM, Meyboom-de-Jong B. 2000. The development of polypharmacy. A longitudinal study. *Family Practice* 17: 261–67.

Zhan C, Sangl J, Bierman AS, et al. 2001. Potentially inappropriate medication use in the community-dwelling elderly. *JAMA* 286: 2823–29.

Useful Links

DrugInfoNet: www.druginfonet.com
Janusinfo: www.janusinfo.org
Pharmacy-related databases: www.pharmacy.org/wwwdbs

Authors
Harriet Finne-Soveri, MD, PhD
Daniela Fialova, PharmD, PhD
Palmi V. Jònsson, MD
Bruce Leff, MD
Gunnar Ljunggren MD, PhD
Knight Steel, MD
Katarzyna Szczerbińska, MD, PhD
Liv Wergeland Sørbye, RN, MA, PhD
Eva Tòpinkova, MD, PhD
John N. Morris, PhD, MSW

Tobacco and Alcohol Use CAP

Problem

The Tobacco and Alcohol Use CAP is concerned with issues related to the consumption of alcohol and the use of tobacco. Excessive consumption of alcohol and any use of tobacco are associated with a variety of unhealthy consequences for persons of any age.

There is strong evidence that any amount of smoking can be harmful to the smoker, as well as to members of the household and health care staff exposed to second-hand smoke. In addition to the well-known risks of cancer and cardiorespiratory disease, tobacco use is an important risk factor for injury (for example, fire, explosion) and reduced quality of life.

Epidemiological studies suggest that small to moderate amounts of alcohol consumption may have beneficial effects. The identification of safe levels of alcohol consumption is a complex problem. Alcohol is less well tolerated by females than males. Some racial groups have especially poor alcohol tolerance.

One drink is defined as the consumption of 0.5 ounces (15 ml) of pure alcohol (ethanol). This amount of ethanol is present in 12 ounces (350 ml) of beer, 5 ounces (140 ml) of wine, or 1.5 ounces (45 ml) of spirits. Dietary guidelines in the United States define moderate drinking in men as no more than two drinks a day and for women as no more than one drink a day.

Background. Smoking is the number one cause of preventable deaths in the world. Approximately 50% of smokers die of a smoking-related illness. The adverse effects of cigarette smoking are more prominent among older adults because of the accumulative injury of many years of exposure. While in younger persons (under 65 years old), the major impact of smoking is an excess risk of cardiovascular disease, the major cause of excess mortality in older adults relates to carcinoma of the lung. Chronic obstructive lung disease (COPD) and cardiovascular disease are also important causes of excess mortality associated with smoking in older persons.

Cessation of smoking is associated with major reductions in the risk of most smoking-related illnesses, even in older adults. Furthermore, cessation of smoking even a few weeks before elective surgery may decrease the risks of the procedure. Older persons are more likely to quit smoking than younger persons, but the benefits of cessation appear to be less powerful, primarily because of previously accumulated effects. Nonetheless, smoking cessation remains the most important method of reducing smoking associated with mortality and morbidity in older persons.

Excess alcohol consumption is often considered to be an issue primarily for younger persons. But disorders related to alcohol are common among older adults and are associated with considerable physical, cognitive, psychological, and social morbidity. Alcohol misuse is more common among men, and socially isolated, single, and separated persons. Older adults are less likely to volunteer information about drinking patterns, and coupled with the perception that alcohol abuse is a problem of younger persons, there is a lower detection rate in older adults. Alcohol excess may present with "atypical" (uncommon) features such as falls, depression, and confusion.

Appropriate levels of alcohol consumption vary by age and sex, although opinions vary among authorities. For example, the National Institute on Alcohol Abuse and Alcoholism (NIAAA) in the United States recommends that persons older than 65 should consume no more than one drink per day. In addition, drug-alcohol interactions and increased potential for accidental injury may be a further concern related to alcohol use among older adults or persons with co-morbid medical or mental health conditions.

Overall Goals of Care

- Ensure that persons who smoke are provided with appropriate advice and support for smoking cessation.

- Offer appropriate advice, support, and treatment to reduce alcohol consumption if indicated and to reduce the risk of harm among persons who consume high levels of alcohol.

Tobacco and Alcohol Use CAP Trigger

This CAP seeks to identify strategies for helping persons cease smoking and cut back on excessive drinking.

TRIGGERED

Persons to whom one or more of the following apply (note that not all of these items appear on every assessment instrument):

- Person feels a need to cut back on drinking or has been told by others to cut down on drinking

- Person who needs a drink first thing in the morning

- Person who has had five or more drinks at a single sitting in the last 14 days

- Daily smoker

This triggered group includes about 10% of persons receiving home care, 5% of persons in long-term care facilities, and 7% of older adults living independently in the community.

NOT TRIGGERED

All other persons.

Tobacco and Alcohol Use CAP Guidelines

Tobacco Use

First, establish the pattern and duration of smoking.

- Consider the current health context. If existing morbidity is associated with smoking (such as ischemic heart disease, stroke, or COPD), there may be a higher level of motivation to quit.

- Consider whether the person lives with a partner who is a nonsmoker — this increases the likelihood of cessation. Mention the partner in the discussions around smoking cessation, but depending on the nature of the relationship, be aware that the dynamics of the relationship may affect smoking behaviors.

- Take into account hazardous situations such as the use of oxygen in the home.

Older adults are more likely to cease smoking, particularly if they indicate that they are motivated. Your efforts will be most fruitful with persons who are in this category.

- The presence of depression may contribute to continuation of smoking, and if there is evidence that it is present, take appropriate measures to further evaluate and manage it. [See Mood CAP.]

Other treatment considerations:

- Advice by itself, is rarely effective.
- In general, some of the most common strategies typically prescribed by physicians are the provision of both counseling and pharmacological agents.
  - Professionals with appropriate training should provide these services.
  - In the case of pharmaceutical agents, the professional must have the authority to prescribe.
  - Nicotine gum, patches, and sprays (Nicotine Replacement Therapy) may be available over the counter in some countries.
  - In general, the combination of counseling and medication appears to produce the best results.

Alcohol Use

First, ascertain the overall pattern of alcohol consumption. This should include current patterns, as well as the lifelong history. This may be a sensitive matter, which may need to be addressed indirectly. There is evidence that many older adults underreport consumption.

The following should lead to an increased emphasis on addressing the drinking problem:

- The person considers a need to reduce the level of drinking.
- Others are concerned about the person's drinking habits.
- The person feels guilty or ashamed about drinking.
- The person sometimes needs a drink first thing in the morning (an "eye-opener").

Information about co-morbid health status may be important. If the person has a number of illnesses, including those affecting cognition, or is taking multiple medications, the level of consumption may need to be minimal or none at all.

- Consider the circumstances that may have created an alcohol-related disorder, for example, bereavement, role changes, or declining health.
- Evaluate the impact of alcohol consumption on the person's health, physical and psychological function, as well as social function.
- If alcohol consumption appears excessive, and particularly if there are associated health problems, medical involvement is essential. Alcohol withdrawal may be associated with serious medical consequences. If a decision to withdraw alcohol is made in a person with a history of heavy consumption, particularly if there are co-morbidities, admission to a hospital for detoxification may be necessary and is recommended by some authorities.

There are two broad presentations of alcohol disorders:

- Lifelong excessive consumption
- Later life increased consumption

Especially if excessive alcohol intake is a recent issue, consider the possibility of depression as a precipitating factor. [See Mood CAP.]

Ascertain the person's perception of the extent of alcohol consumption and motivation to curtail (cut back) consumption. Persons with addictions to tobacco, alcohol, or other substances may be at different stages of readiness for change. For example, some may be unaware of their problem or have never considered changing their behavior. They may not be prepared to consider any changes to their current health behaviors. Others may be thinking about changing their use of these substances. Consequently, they may be more open to receiving information about treatment options and support programs.

Potential interventions:

- Short-term inpatient treatment may be necessary for detoxification or to deal with withdrawal symptoms.

- Psychotropic medications may be useful, although care must be taken in their use with older adults.

- Group therapy is a frequently used treatment. It creates opportunities to enhance self-image, share anxieties, and restore the ability to enter into relationships. Older alcoholics participating in group treatment tend to fare better when the group is age-specific. Some anecdotal evidence also suggests that the most successful groups may be gender-specific.

- Alcohol dependency, especially for early-onset alcoholics, is a chronic disease from which recovery is often a long-term process.

- Referral to a substance abuse professional, especially one with experience with geriatric patients, may be useful.

- As in all substance abuse treatment, often the involvement of family and the person's support network in the treatment process may be critical. Indeed, the intervention may have to be focused at least initially on the effect on the family. This is necessary not only for the treatment of the person, but also because family members may be suffering from serious psychological and sometimes physical trauma as a result of the person's behavior.

Additional Resources

Burns DM. 2000. Cigarette smoking among the elderly: Disease consequences and the benefits of cessation. *Am J Health Promot* 14(6): 357–61.

Dale LC, Olsen DA, Patten CA, et al. 1997. Predictors of smoking cessation among elderly smokers treated for nicotine dependence. *Tobacco Control* 6(3): 181–87.

O'Connell H, Chin AV, Cunningham C, Lawlor B. 2003. Alcohol use disorders in elderly people — redefining an age old problem in old age. *BMJ* 327(7416): 664–67.

Prochaska JO, DiClemente CC, Norcross JC. 1992. In search of how people change: Applications to addictive behaviors. *Am Psychol* 47(9): 1102–14.

Ranney L, Melvin C, Lux L, McClain E, Lohr KN. 2006. Systematic review: Smoking cessation intervention strategies for adults and adults in special populations. *Ann Intern Med* 145(11): 845–56.

Authors

Len Gray, MD, PhD
John P. Hirdes, PhD
Charles Phillips, PhD, MPH
Knight Steel, MD

Urinary Incontinence CAP

Problem

Urinary incontinence is the inability to control urine in a socially appropriate manner. In the United States, 15% of older adults living at home have a urinary incontinence problem. In long-term care facilities, over 50% of persons experience urinary incontinence either occasionally or on a regular basis. This problem is often cited as a factor in the decision to move from a home environment to an assisted living facility or a long-term care facility.

Although it frequently increases with age, urinary incontinence is not a normal part of the biological process of aging. Regrettably, it is often embarrassing and therefore not even mentioned to the health care provider. Discussing the problem openly with the person and family members is the first step in developing a successful plan of care.

Urinary incontinence causes many problems, including skin rashes, falls, isolation, pressure ulcers, and the potentially troubling use of indwelling catheters. Catheter use increases the risk of life-threatening infections. Use of catheters also contributes to discomfort and the needless use of medications that are often required for the treatment of the associated bladder spasms.

Overall Goals of Care

- Recognize urinary incontinence and establish the cause.

- Expedite improvement in bladder function in those who could improve by instituting appropriate diagnostic and therapeutic interventions.

- Prevent increasing degrees of incontinence in persons who are already incontinent and may benefit from a treatment program.

Urinary Incontinence CAP Trigger

The goal of this CAP is first to expedite improvement in bladder function in those who could so improve, and second, to prevent worsening of bladder function in persons who may have the ability to respond to a treatment program. The following rules indicate the two subgroups of persons triggered for specialized follow-up, as well as the two subgroups that are not targeted for follow-up.

TRIGGERED TO FACILITATE IMPROVEMENT IN BLADDER FUNCTION

Included in this group are persons who have **all** of the following characteristics:

- Have reoccurring episodes of incontinence (even if less than weekly) or no urine output.

- Have at least a minimal level of cognitive abilities (as indicated by being Independent or having Modified Independence in Cognitive Skills for Daily Decision Making).

- Not totally dependent or receiving extensive assistance in locomotion, and

- Have **either or both** of the following acute triggering criteria:

  - **Not** on a scheduled toileting program

  - One or more of the following indicators are present that suggest the person is in a fluctuating status, and thus his or her urinary incontinence may be of more recent onset, or subject to improvement:

    - Hip fracture
    - Recent decline in ADLs
    - Use of an indwelling catheter
    - Pneumonia
    - Diarrhea

This group includes about 5% of persons in long-term care facilities, 10% of persons receiving home care, and 2% of older adults living independently in the community. In a long-term care facility setting, about 22% of the persons triggered into this group will improve over a 90-day period. The rate of improvement in home care is about the same, at 16%. At the same time, however, some in this group will decline over 90 days; in long-term care facilities about 15% will decline and in home care about 10% will decline.

TRIGGERED TO PREVENT DECLINE — Higher Rate of Decline Expected

Included in this group are persons who have **all** of the following characteristics:

- Reoccurring episodes of incontinence (even if less than weekly) or no urine output.

- Independent to Moderately Impaired in Cognitive Skills for Daily Decision Making (thus they are not Severely Impaired).

- **Do not** meet the two **above** acute criteria under the Improvement Trigger (the scheduled toileting program and the fluctuating status criteria).

This group includes about 40% of persons in long-term care facilities, 24% of persons receiving home care, and 5% of older adults living independently in the community. In a long-term care facility setting, about 20% of the persons triggered into this group will decline over a 90-day period, while 10% will improve. The rate of decline in home care is about 10%, while the improvement rate is also about 10%.

NOT TRIGGERED — Continent

This group consists of those who are continent at the time of assessment.

This group includes about 35% of persons in long-term care facilities, 55% of persons receiving home care, and 92% of older adults living independently in the community. In a long-term care facility setting, about 13% of the persons triggered into this group will decline over a 90-day period. The rate of decline in home care is about 11%.

NOT TRIGGERED — Poor Decision Making

This group is assessed as Severely Impaired (or having no discernable consciousness) for Cognitive Skills for Daily Decision Making at the time of assessment.

This group includes about 15% of persons in long-term care facilities, 11% of persons receiving home care, and less than 1% of older adults living independently in the community. In a long-term care facility setting, about 26% of the persons triggered into this group will decline over a 90-day period, while 4% will improve. In home care the rate of decline is about 20%, while the improvement rate is about 8%.

Urinary incontinence is the inability to control urine in a socially appropriate manner, and for many this means the person cannot hold his or her urine until he or she reaches a toilet. There are multiple classifications of incontinence, the common causes being grouped into five general categories: stress, urge, mixed (stress and urge), overflow, and functional. There are a number of causes of each (see the following), and there are considerable differences between men and women in the likelihood of each type. To a great extent this reflects differences in the length of the urethra, the tube exiting the bladder, and in women who have experienced pregnancy or childbirth, changes in the anatomy of the pelvis. In addition, many older adults are incontinent because they simply cannot make it to the bathroom in time, for example, those who have limitations in ambulation because of arthritis or a stroke.

Types of Incontinence

Stress incontinence. Incontinence that occurs during coughing, sneezing, laughing, lifting heavy objects, or making other movements that put pressure or stress on the bladder. Leakage tends to be of small amounts of urine with the stimulus. In some reports this condition is the most common form of incontinence in women, resulting from weak pelvic muscles or a weakening of the wall between the bladder and the vagina. In women, the weakness is commonly due to pregnancy and childbirth or lower levels of the hormone estrogen during menstrual periods or after menopause. In men, stress incontinence may occur postprostatectomy. Often stress incontinence is eliminated or markedly reduced in frequency by

- Pelvic floor muscle rehabilitation, for which there is strong evidence of effectiveness for persons with stress incontinence. This should be the first line of treatment offered.

- Lifestyle counseling to encourage appropriate amounts of fluid, limited alcohol and caffeinated drinks, and weight loss for overweight persons.

- Medications may be prescribed by a physician to be used in combination with pelvic floor strengthening exercises, but the drugs may have side effects.

- Biofeedback, acupuncture, and electrical stimulation have been used in conjunction with pelvic floor reeducation programs with varying levels of effectiveness.

- Intravaginal devices, for example, pessaries

- Implants

- Surgery

Urge incontinence (also called overactive or spastic bladder). An unplanned loss of urine after feeling a sudden urge to urinate such as while sleeping, drinking water, or listening to water running. Leakage tends to be of significant amounts of urine with each episode. Treatments for urge incontinence include

- Biofeedback

- Timed voiding

- Bladder training

- Medications such as anticholinergics and antispasmotics to relax muscles and block nerve signals leading to bladder spasms

Mixed incontinence. Involuntary leakage associated with urgency and also with exertion, effort, sneezing, or coughing. The predominant condition, stress or urge incontinence, should be treated first.

Overflow incontinence. Incontinence that occurs when the bladder is constantly full and reaches a point where it overflows and leaks urine. This condition can occur when the urethra is blocked due to causes such as urinary stones, tumors, or an enlarged prostate. It may also be the result of weak bladder muscles, due to nerve damage from diabetes or other diseases. This is a common form of incontinence in men. Treatment may involve

- Timed voiding

- Bladder training

- Intermittent catheterization

- Medication such as those listed below have been prescribed by physicians to improve urine flow or shrink the prostate:

  - Alpha blockers are used to treat problems caused by prostate enlargement and bladder outlet obstruction.

  - Medications such as alpha reductase inhibitors have been prescribed to shrink an enlarged prostate.

- Surgery and radiation

Functional incontinence. A loss of urine in a person whose urinary tract function is such that he or she should be able to maintain continence, but who because of physical disabilities, external obstacles, or problems in thinking or communicating is unable to get to the bathroom before urinating. Eliminating or reducing the functional incontinence depends on identifying and treating the underlying problem. [See ADL CAP to improve mobility and transfers.]

Incontinence Assessment

There are multiple factors that cause or contribute to incontinence. Identifying and improving these factors can improve continence. It is important to be aware of risk factors for incontinence in order to raise the topic, as it is sometimes difficult for persons to discuss continence issues. Risk factors include age, childhood problems such as bedwetting, prostatectomy in men, and pregnancy and childbirth in women. High Body Mass Index (BMI) is also a risk factor. Menopause is a contributing factor in women.

It is important to obtain a good history and description of the problem, with the goal of determining whether the incontinence is transient or established in character. The description can include information from standardized tests of function and symptoms, a urinary diary (detailing the times and amount of incontinence as well as the circumstances — for example, when coughing, and the amount of urine voided when the person does reach the bathroom), and stress tests such as coughing to see if they elicit incontinence.

Testing methods include the following:

- Physical exam (includes pelvic and rectal exams)

- Stress testing (for example, having a woman cough and see if there is leakage of urine)

- Observation of voiding or uroflometer (looking for stream size, hesitation, volume of urine)

- Urinalysis

- Urine culture

- Evaluation of postvoid residual urine is an important diagnostic parameter that should be considered in persons with complex histories.

- Cystoscopy

- Urodynamic evaluation

Modifiable factors contributing to transitory urinary incontinence are listed below, and they can be addressed to improve continence. Treatable underlying factors that should be routinely "ruled out" are presented under the acronym "DIAPPERS."

Delirium

Infection (UTI)

Atrophic vaginitis

Pharmaceuticals/Medications (of many types)

Psychological and psychiatric problems

Excessive urine output

Restricted mobility

Stool constipation/impaction

The following are potential underlying causes of incontinence that can be addressed to improve continence:

- **Delirium** — Identify cause of delirium, including recent hospitalizations as well as pharmaceutical agents. [See Delirium CAP.]

- **Infection (UTI)** — A symptomatic urinary tract infection (blood in urine, frequency of urination, urge, burning on urination, WBC elevation in urinalysis). Refer for further medical examination to include urinalysis, culture, and course of antibiotics.

- **Atrophic vaginitis** — These conditions in postmenopausal women often cause lower urinary tract symptoms. Use of appropriate creams or the use of an estrogen ring may be helpful.

- **Atrophic urethritis** — This condition leads to thinning of the lining of the urethra, causing local irritation and loss of the mucosal seal. Incontinence due to atrophic urethritis is often characterized by urgency and dysuria (painful urination).

- **Pharmaceuticals/Medications** — Medications may cause persons to have transient incontinence, but they may also be useful in improving incontinence. It is helpful to review the person's medications for potential effects on incontinence as well as to search the literature for new medications that may be helpful. Alcohol use and medication use are common causes of transient incontinence in older adults. [See Appropriate Medications CAP, as well as Tobacco and Alcohol CAP.]

  - Diuretics ("fluid pills" taken to reduce blood pressure, or for CHF) can lead to sudden onset of urge incontinence.

  - Anticholinergics can lead to overflow incontinence (these medications cause the bladder not to contract, the bladder becomes full, and urine leaks out).

  - Nighttime incontinence can be caused or exacerbated by heart failure, peripheral venous insufficiency, and medications. Before altering a person's medication, a physician must be contacted.

■ **Psychological and psychiatric problems** — Severe depression. [See Mood CAP.]

   ▪ Initial treatment focuses on depression.

■ **Excessive urine output** — This condition can be caused by high fluid intake (including alcohol and caffeine). The person should be encouraged to adjust his or her fluid intake to produce a 24-hour urinary output of between 1,000 ml and 2,000 ml.

■ **Restricted mobility** — This can prevent a person from reaching the toilet in time and may result from physical limitations, inability to get out of a bed or chair independently, impaired vision, fear of falling, or foot problems. [See ADL CAP for suggestions on improving mobility and Physical Activities Promotion CAP for suggestions on exercise.]

   ▪ Consider environmental adaptations — for example, offering mobility aids, facilitating entry to the bathroom, placing a commode near the bed at night, and instituting an assisted toileting program.

■ **Stool constipation/impaction** — Presence of constipation may lead to an impaction (a mass of hardened stool stuck in the intestinal tract). Presence of a fecal impaction may lead to pressure or stimulation of the bladder. Usually these persons have urge or overflow incontinence. Removing the impaction should restore continence.

Appliances and Pads

Factors to Consider for Brief/Pad Use:

- Fit

- Cost

- Absorbency

- Gender of the user

- Activity level of the user (person mostly sits all day, or person walks around and changes position more frequently)

- Ability of the user to insert and remove brief/pad

- Ability of the user to clean/launder brief-type garments

- Ability of the user to handle disposable pad waste

What to Use:

- There is no one-size-fits-all brief/pad.

- It is best to try a small quantity of a few different types/brands of pads/briefs.

- Pads placed on chairs are not very useful for an active person. Also, they are very noticeable.

Additional Resources

Balmforth JR, Mantle J, Bidmead J, Cardozo L. 2006. A prospective observational trial of pelvic floor muscle training for female stress urinary incontinence. *BJU Int.* (October) 98(4): 811–17.

European Association of Urology: www.uroweb.org.

National Institute for Health and Clinical Excellence. 2007. NICE Guideline 50, Urinary incontinence. National Collaborating Center for Acute Care, London, England. www.nice.org.uk

NAFC: National Association for Continence; www.nacf.org. 1-800-BLADDER; 1-800-252-3337

National Institutes of Health: www.nih.gov; including the AGE Pages: www.niapublications.org/shopagepages

SIGN: Scottish Incontinence Guidelines Network. Management of Urinary Incontinence in Primary Care. www.sign.ac.uk/pdf/sign79.pdf

Urinary incontinence: 2005. *Clinical Practice Guideline,* AMDA.

Wainner, RS. 2005. Urinary incontinence is no longer just your grandmother's concern. www.texpts.com/uplimg/UINotJustGrandmotherProblem.pdf

Authors

Pauline Belleville-Taylor, RN, MS, CS
Knight Steel, MD
Katherine Berg, PhD, PT
John N. Morris, PhD, MSW

Bowel Conditions CAP

Problem

The Bowel Conditions CAP addresses three of the most common bowel conditions seen in older adults and disabled adults: constipation, diarrhea, and fecal incontinence.

A standard definition of constipation does not exist. Perhaps most commonly it is defined in the literature as not having a bowel movement for 3 or more days. If a person does not have a bowel movement for this period of time, usually the stool is harder than normal and may be difficult to expel. Some persons have hard stools or find it uncomfortable to have a bowel movement even if the frequency is daily. Such persons usually tell their physician that they are constipated. Constipation accounts for about 2.5 million physician visits per year. The prevalence of constipation in older persons living in the community is about 20%. Its high prevalence in older adults likely reflects in part changes in the colon associated with the aging process.

Diarrhea may refer to frequent bowel movements and/or to loose or watery stools. This condition, like the others, may be chronic or acute. Often it is associated with abdominal pain, fever, or other symptoms. Diarrhea may be just mildly annoying or life threatening. It may be caused by an acute infectious agent or may reflect a disease especially of the colon (for example, diverticulitis) or the small intestine. It may also be noted when the person's colon is impacted with stool and only loose stool is expelled.

Isolated fecal incontinence may be a rare occurrence. Often it is associated with one of the two previous complaints or it may be a chronic and exceptionally difficult issue to manage. On occasion it may reflect damage to the anal sphincter, especially if it is a frequent occurrence. It is especially of concern to many because of its impact on social functioning.

Overall Goals of Care

- Recognize the existence of one or more of these three conditions and establish a cause for its existence.
- Address each in such a way that the person is able to function as normally as possible.
- Be able to monitor bowel function over time.

27

The goal of this CAP is twofold: first, to facilitate improvement in bowel status whenever possible; and second, to prevent avoidable bowel decline. To identify these triggered groups, one must first calculate two risk summaries (decline and improvement).

- First, count the number of the following **Risk of Decline** criteria:

  - Cognitive Skills for Daily Decision Making (Severely Impaired);

  - Eating (Supervision through Total Dependence);

  - Bed mobility (Total Dependence, Did not occur);

  - Bladder continence (Incontinent);

  - Easily distracted (Behavior different);

  - Periods of altered perceptions or awareness of surroundings (Behavior different);

  - Episodes of disorganized speech (Behavior different);

  - Mental function varies over the course of the day (Behavior different).

- Second, count the number of the following **Risk of Improvement** items:

  - Toilet use (Independent through Limited Assistance);

  - Formal caregivers and direct care staff believe the person is capable of increased independence;

  - Pneumonia;

  - Deteriorated;

  - Bladder continence (Continent and Usually continent);

  - Hip fracture in the last 180 days.

TRIGGERED TO FACILITATE IMPROVEMENT

All of the following must be present:

- Risk of Decline count (from previous section) equal to 0 or 1, **and**

- Risk of Improvement count (from previous section) equal to 2 or higher, **and**

- Bowel continence: Infrequently incontinent to Incontinent

This group includes about 5% of persons in long-term care facilities, 7% of persons receiving home care, and less than 1% of older adults living independently in the community. In a long-term care facility setting, about 33% of the persons triggered into this group will improve over a 90-day period (while 19% will decline); the rate of improvement in home care is about 20% (while 6% will decline).

TRIGGERED TO PREVENT DECLINE

All of the following must be present:

- Risk of Decline count (from previous section) equal to 2 or higher, **and**

- Bowel continence: Not fully incontinent

This group includes about 15% of persons in long-term care facilities, 6% of persons receiving home care, and less than 1% of older adults living independently in the community. In a long-term care facility setting, about 30% of the persons triggered into this group will decline over a 90-day period (while 11% will improve); the rate of decline in home care is about 14% (while 13% will improve).

NOT TRIGGERED   All other persons. Some of these persons have bowel problems at the time of assessment, and would receive normal care for bowel problems when present.

Bowel Conditions CAP Guidelines

Assessment and Care Planning

A person having any of these conditions must be evaluated to determine the duration of the symptom, its severity, and the presence of any other complaints. Look for indications of malaise, abdominal pain, fever, or the presence of blood in the stool or dark stools (which may reflect bleeding higher up in the GI tract). All persons with a significant change in bowel habits, fever, blood in the stool, associated pain, or persistent abnormalities require medical evaluation.

One or more of these three conditions may reflect a decline in mobility, a recent change in diet, the introduction of a new medication, decreased fluid intake (for any reason), or even excessive environmental heat.

Once the cause is determined, the key concern for optimal care planning is the promotion of a pattern of bowel function such that the person does not experience discomfort or any social inconvenience.

Bowel Problem Assessment

What is the history of the problem?

- How many bowel movements did the person have within the last few days? Is this pattern "normal" for the person? What was the consistency of the stool?

- Was there evidence of blood in the stool (either red stool or unusually dark stool)?

- If there was incontinence, was it a large amount of stool, or just a small amount? Was the person fully aware of the passage of the stool?

- Is there a history of anorectal or colonic surgery, or in a female, damage to the rectum at the time of delivery?

- Is there a history of intolerance to certain foods, especially milk?

- Has the person passed excessive amounts of gas or felt bloated?

- Did the person have a fever or experience malaise?

- Did the person vomit or have abdominal pain?

- Is there a recent change in the person's diet, fiber, or fluid intake?

- Does the person have a known condition, such as diverticulosis or diabetes, that might help explain the symptoms?

- What medications is the person taking? Have any new medications been started recently?

- Is there a history of laxative use and, if so, has it been excessive?

What are the characteristics of the stool?

- Description of stool type: consistency, color, unusual odors, presence of frank blood.

- Is the person straining when he or she tries to defecate?

- Does the person have pain associated with bowel movements?

What are the characteristics of the bowel pattern?

- Does the person have a pattern for moving his or her bowels?

- Is it different recently?

- Does the person need to share a bathroom, or is he or she otherwise not assured of privacy when using the toilet?

Care Planning Suggestions

Care plan suggestions for persons with constipation. Strategies for improving diet, activity, and bowel pattern can be woven into the daily life of the person.

- Especially if of recent onset, evaluation by a physician is indicated to rule out a colonic tumor or other such cause.

- Identify the person's bowel pattern. Record the person's bowel movements and ask about his or her bowel habits. If fecal impaction is indicated it may be necessary to perform a rectal exam to determine the presence of stool in the rectum.

- Identify the presence of hemorrhoids or anal fissures. Consult a physician and provide topical anesthetics as needed.

- Assess the person for the presence of dementia or depression. Persons with depression need to be referred for mental health services. Persons with a dementia will benefit from a habit-training or bowel-training program.

- Ask about the person's medications and any laxative or enema use. Anticholinergics, narcotics, calcium channel blockers, some incontinence medications, iron, diuretics, tranquilizers, and antacids can cause constipation. Excessive use of laxatives and enemas can increase problems with constipation.

- Ask about the person's daily diet. Provide fluids and encourage the person to increase fluid intake. Increasing fiber intake should be done slowly over a matter of a few weeks to a month.

- Encourage toileting opportunities. Provide a bedside commode or an elevated toilet seat. Remind the person to go to the toilet after breakfast, or after a meal, or whenever the person is most likely to move his or her bowels.

- Provide opportunities for the person to increase daily physical activity. Regular walking and other physical activities can help to decrease or eliminate constipation.

Care plan suggestions for persons with fecal incontinence:

- Referral to a physician is indicated especially if onset is recent or associated with blood in the stool.

- Encourage the person to have bowel evacuation at the same time each day.

- Determine the presence of neuromuscular weakness. Persons with this problem may benefit from elimination training. Administer a suppository 30 minutes prior to scheduled elimination.

- Establish and monitor a bowel regimen that includes fluids, diet modification, scheduling, stool softener, suppository, and digital stimulation.

- Assess for the presence of fecal impaction. Remove impaction if present.

- For persons with chronic diarrhea as the cause of fecal incontinence, the physician may prescribe loperamide as a helpful medication.

- For fecal incontinence due to rectal sphincter disturbances, biofeedback may be effective.

- Meticulous skin care is a priority after episodes of fecal incontinence.

- At times, it may be necessary to use pads or briefs.

Care plan suggestions for persons with diarrhea:

- If severe, acute, or associated with pain, blood in the stool, or fever, immediate medical referral is indicated.

- Has the person recently been started on a new medication?

- Has the person recently started tube feedings? Dilute the feedings or change the rate of feeding.

- Is lactose intolerance suspected? Remove all sources of lactose from the diet.

- Is an intestinal bacterial infection suspected? Obtain a stool specimen for analysis.

- Is a fecal impaction suspected? Obtain an abdominal flat plate x-ray. Remove fecal impaction if present.

- Provide plenty of fluids that are noncarbonated and nondairy. When diarrhea is persistent or present with vomiting, dehydration may soon follow.

- Is lactose intolerance suspected? Remove all sources of lactose from the diet.

- Is an intestinal bacterial infection suspected? Obtain a stool specimen for analysis.

- Medications for diarrhea:

    - For nonspecific diarrhea, the physician may prescribe treatment with psyllium, methylcellulose, or loperamide.

    - For infectious diarrhea, therapy is targeted to suspected or identified pathogens.

- Meticulous skin care is a priority after episodes of diarrhea.

Consideration of further evaluation:

- Once the existence of constipation, diarrhea, or fecal incontinence has been established, it will be necessary to determine whether further testing is required.

- In the person with an abrupt onset of severe diarrhea who had been taking antibiotics recently (for another reason), a stool culture and a test for the toxins of C difficile would be indicated.

- If the person is having crampy abdominal pain and even mild diarrhea, he or she might require a CT scan to rule out diverticulitis or other conditions.

- If blood, either red or black, has been noted, this usually requires further evaluation such as a colonoscopic study and perhaps studies of the esophagus, stomach, and small intestine as well.

- In a large number of persons, the problem is chronic and appropriate interventions can be implemented.

Additional Resources

American Medical Directors Association. 2006. Clinical practice guidelines: Gastrointestinal disorders in the long-term care setting. Columbia, MD.

Carpenito-Moyet L. 2004. *Nursing care plans and documentation*, 4th ed. Philadelphia, PA: Lippincott, Williams & Wilkins.

Finne-Soveri H, Sorbye LW, Jonsson PV, Carpenter GI, Bernabei R. 2007. Increased work-load associated with fecal incontinence among home care patients in 11 European countries. Accepted for publication in the *European Journal of Public Health*.

McGough Monks K. 2003. *Gastrointestinal system assessment in home health nursing.* St. Louis, MO: Mosby.

National Digestive Diseases Information Clearinghouse (NDDIC), Bethesda, MD: www.digestive.niddk.nih.gov/about/contact.htm

National Institute for Health and Clinical Excellence. 2007. NICE Guideline 49, Faecal incontinence. National Collaborating Center for Acute Care, London, England: www.nice.org.uk

Authors

Pauline Belleville-Taylor, RN, MS, CS
Knight Steel, MD
John N. Morris, PhD, MSW

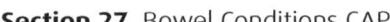

List of Abbreviations

AC	Acute Care
ADL	Activities of Daily Living
AL	Assisted Living
ATC	anatomical therapeutic chemical
BUN	blood urea nitrogen
CA	Contact Assessment
CAPs	Clinical Assessment Protocols
CF	Mental Health for Correctional Facilities
CHA	Community Health Assessment
CMH	Community Mental Health
CVA	cerebrovascular accident
ESP	Emergency Screener for Psychiatry
GI	gastrointestinal
GU	genitourinary
HC	Home Care
IADL	Instrumental Activities of Daily Living
ICD-CM	International Classification of Diseases, Clinical Modification
ID	Intellectual Disability
LTCF	Long-Term Care Facilities
MDS	Minimum Data Set
MH	Mental Health
NDC	National Drug Code
PAC	Post-Acute Care
PC	Palliative Care
PRN	pro re nata ("as needed")
QOL	Self-Report Quality of Life
RAI	Resident Assessment Instrument
RUGs	Resource Utilization Groups
TENS	transcutaneous electrical nerve stimulation
WELL	Wellness

CPSIA information can be obtained at www.ICGtesting.com
Printed in the USA
LVOW01s1931250214

374987LV00006B/14/P